Healing
with Chakra
Energy

Healing with Chakra Energy

Restoring the Natural Harmony of the Body

Lilla Bek and Philippa Pullar

Destiny Books
Rochester, Vermont

Destiny Books
One Park Street
Rochester, Vermont 05767

LIBRARY OF CONGRESS CATALOGING-IN-PUBLICATION DATA

Bek, Lilla.
    Healing with Chakra energy : restoring the natural harmony of the
body / Lilla Bek and Philippa Pullar.
        p.   cm.
    Originally published in 1986 under title: The seven levels of healing.
    Includes index.
    ISBN 0-89281-513-2
    1. Mental healing. 2. Chakras. I. Pullar, Philippa, 1935–
II. Title.
    RZ401.B355 1995
    615.8'52--dc20   94–12262
                                          CIP

Printed and bound in the United States

10 9 8 7 6 5 4 3 2

Destiny Books is a division of Inner Traditions International

Distributed to the book trade in Canada by Publishers Group West (PGW), Toronto, Ontario

Contents

Foreword by Don Copland

When I first met Lilla Bek several years ago, through our mutual interest in spiritual healing, it did not take long for me to realise that behind her quiet, gentle and unassuming exterior lay an inner depth of immense wisdom. I was soon to discover that she was no ordinary person. Extraordinary is more accurate! The incredible flow of knowledge emanating through Lilla's consciousness could only be shared initially by those students fortunate enough to attend one of her courses. With the advent of this book, *The Seven Levels of Healing*, everyone who is interested in healing and the healing process can gain a deeper understanding of the processes involved.

Healers must always be prepared to accept responsibility for their work and to act as ambassadors for spiritual healing. They can only do this if they are able to understand the energies that are available and from which level they are using these energies when they are acting as an instrument.

It is not surprising, in such a sick society as confronts us now, that more and more interest is being shown in the ancient art of spiritual healing. Accompanying this tendency is a proliferation of therapists using many forms of healing. Sadly, some of the techniques being used do not acknowledge a spiritual base and some therapists seem unaware that the whole point of healing is to enable a person to get in touch with their inner self and to create a situation in which the healing is totally holistic, including spiritual benefit as well.

Without it the patient is deprived of the deeper meaning of life which in itself is very often the cause of the illness.

A spiritual healer is creating a possibility for the patient to become linked with the origin and essence of the spiritual force rather than manipulating with that force, without comprehending its great depth. Healers need a great deal of compassion, a depth of love and peace, but they should also seek to develop their own personal harmony and attunement to enable them to operate from the highest possible level of awareness within their reach. All the tools for assisting the healer in this endeavour may be found in this book which contains exercises and suggestions for the reader to expand and develop.

The National Federation of Spiritual Healers is the main national and international non-denominational healing organization for spiritual healers and has a membership of 4000. The word 'spiritual' in its title refers to the acknowl- edged divine source of energy and to that responsive element in Man seen by healers as comprised of body, mind and spirit. The NFSH presents training and development courses which are designed to direct, assist and perhaps accelerate the development of the potential healer to become a safe and spiritual channel through which these energies can flow. All the advanced courses are taken by Lilla Bek and examine the deeper aspects of healing. Preceding these are basic devel- opment courses which over the past few years have been attended by people from all walks of life, including many of the caring professions such as doctors, dentists, social workers, probation officers, nurses, medical students and others. Many of the subjects mentioned in this book form part of the Federation's syllabus. Students are reminded that spiritual healing is the art and science of assisting in the restoration of the patient's health, at all levels of Man's being, irrespective of where, in the body, ill health may have manifested. By the laying on of hands, by attunement through prayer and meditation – whether in the presence of the patient or not – a healer seeks to induce a beneficial effect upon the patient's life-force at all levels of consciousness. Ultimately, the healer acts as a catalyst in order to strengthen the patient sufficiently to make beneficial changes in his own lifestyle, supported by love and the healing energies involved.

All the main healing organizations cooperate within the Confederation of Healing Organisations and they have achieved a common code of conduct and insurance cover for all their probationers and healers. Within these rules spiritual healing, in relation to orthodox medicine, is complementary rather than alternative and healers' advice in no way counteracts that of the patient's doctor. The CHO has undertaken a five-year project of medical research supervised by independent medical experts. This research programme is designed to include the treatment by spiritual healing of six specific illnesses, the research being carried out on selected patients in selected areas At the time of writing the first study undertaken was for cataracts closely followed by one for NHS hospital out-patients in Yorkshire with rheumatoid arthritis. The objective is to persuade the medical profession to accept healing as a therapy to be used in conjunction with orthodox methods. Most people are unaware that healing is officially listed as a therapy within the NHS and, although a few doctors do prescribe it, this by no means normal practice.

In order to reach his full potential, the healer must increase his awareness of the enormity of his task within his work. This book brings to light the fact that the healer not only has a great responsibility to his patient but also to God and His Law. The healer is a mediator between heaven and earth, a junction point between spirit and physical matter.

The physical form of Man is but a temporary dwelling house for the spirit as it gains further experience in the world of matter. With knowledge Man can confidently allow his consciousness to rise to higher levels and realize that the way to final freedom is through the self in understanding and love – this is self-healing in its widest sense.

To have understanding the healer must have knowledge of the energies he is channelling. *The Seven Levels of Healing* provides this knowledge in great detail. It shows us the tapestry of the universe itself, the tapestry within which we weave our own individual pattern which forms part of the whole.

I feel confident that the reader of this book who is truly

seeking to understand himself more fully and to make himself more whole cannot help but find much to intrigue and to encourage him along this path.

Introduction

In this, so-called, New Age there is much interest in learning to develop the natural healing gifts. This book is for all who are interested in spiritual healing. It explains what it is and how it works. Although written basically for those seeking to augment their own healing ability, it is also for people who want to know more about the subject, in general, and self-healing in particular. After all, any healing process is essentially self-healing, no one really cures anyone else; all they can do is to help the patient to heal himself. Doctors are recognizing more and more the crucial role the mind plays in health. In any case it is always beneficial to have the patient's cooperation during the healing endeavour no matter what system of medicine is being employed. Spiritual healing is certainly no exception to this rule.

The first thing to make clear is that spiritual healing is not the same thing as Spiritualism. Many people believe that spiritual healing is something weird, with apparitions and spirits manifesting all over the place. This is not the case. There is nothing eerie about spiritual healing and one of the aims of this book is to dispel any mystery surrounding the subject.

In order, then, to understand what is widely meant by the term 'spiritual healing' let us first look at the following remark: 'Mr X will not live: he has lost his spirit.' Let us see what this implies. It suggests that there is an animation inside Mr X which goes beyond his physical body and his mind. It suggests that Mr X, together with all human beings, have within them a feeling of continuity, an essence which is linked to a source, an awareness of origin. Spiritual healing aims to connect to this well-head. It does not just make the patient physically better, it works to bring him back to his own source, his own inner peace, his own creativity. You could put it another way and say that spiritual healing returns the body to its roots, takes it home so that it can heal and restore itself.

This brings us to the question of religion. Is it possible to be a spiritual healer, people ask, without being religious? In one sense all spiritual healers are religious but in a very practical way. They are not attempting to impose external beliefs on people but rather trying to help them be healthy by bringing them closer to the creative potential inside themselves. Spiritual healing is not faith healing. Neither the healer nor his patient necessarily needs to be of a particular persuasion. After all, a human body can replenish itself and its cells can be reborn, regardless of whether or not its owner believes in a creator. Certainly some people can find peace without following any religion and they can be loving, gentle and kind without believing in God. It is ultimately the healer's ability to channel energy which is crucial. Many do hold that Christ is healing through them; many work with the understanding that the whole of humanity is under the guardianship of a higher being which we can call what we like – God, cosmic consciousness and so on. But again some believe in very little. Certain types of healing are effective regardless of faith. It is possible to heal just through using techniques, as we shall see. What is essential to the healing process is a conviction about *something*. Everyone needs some kind of project in their mind, something they can continue to do. If they do not have this there will be nothing to live for, they lose their will to live: in other words, they lose their spirit. This is borne out by the research of certain insurance companies which reveals that a large percentage of men die just two or three years after retirement. With no job they lose their sense of continuity, they have no project towards which to direct their attention and they lose their will to live.

So now we come to the healing energy itself. This is the same vital force which can be directed, among other things, to making money, to creating a successful career, composing works of art, even to the pursuit of pleasure. It is through

12

channelling this vital flux that it is possible to heal others. Everybody has this vital energy with the potential for conducting it in order to restore others, but most of us are not aware that it is composed of different levels and we have to discover with which of these we are dealing. The highest levels of healing are linked to the essence of genius. An inspired artist who creates a fine painting will go beyond the limits of that which people can generally produce; it is the same with a healer. In other words, there is a level at which things come through us rather than from our experience, from what we have gathered and learnt.

Healing is a gift, then, which many people have. Most mothers can soothe their children by putting their hands on them to alleviate their hurts, their cuts and bruises. Many people have the gift but not in a complete way and they do not understand the mechanics of it. For instance, some very passive people are naturally healing and calming. By their very presence they initiate stillness in others and help them to get better. Another type can be inspiring, stirring their companions to various forms of creativity and producing in them a transcendence. So it is possible to help by being passive and it is equally possible to heal by being active. In between there is another possibility, which is neither active nor passive. Such healers get rid of themselves, as it were, and simply act as channels.

So healing can occur on many levels according not only to the healer's awareness and his ability to channel energy but also to the receptivity of his patient. Of course there are some people who are better at doing it than others. This is true of anything, whether it be painting, making love or even cooking. All of these can create a feeling of expansion and well-being, they can be healing and beautiful and, in the hands of a master, they can, when carried out on the highest levels, lead to transcendental experiences.

Perhaps the simplest way to describe healing is as an exchange of energies, a reaction between two people. Success depends just as much on the receiving as on the giving. In other words, unless the patient is receptive, unless a rapport can be established, the healing will not really work. Imagine a love affair or giving a party. These are both exchanges of energy on different levels and depend for their success on the quality of giving and the quality of receiving. One-sided affairs are not made in heaven, nor are parties where the guests are unable to communicate or the hosts have failed to provide adequate warmth and hospitality.

Before Philippa turned to healing she used to entertain a lot. She must have enjoyed making houses beautiful, cooking and putting people at their ease. Usually the parties were successful and, at the time, a certain energy, a certain expansion and warmth were generated. Yet it struck her how inadequate this sort of exchange really was. On the whole it ended in nothing but exhaustion, to say nothing of hangovers, as ideas were batted backwards and forwards over the table and the wine sank down in the bottle. This was dissipating energy rather than creating it. It struck her, too, how inadequate this was to help people when they were depressed, seriously ill or dying. Words were often of little use. When eventually she became involved in healing she found this exchange, often taking place as it did in silence, much more refreshing and supportive, both in the giving and the receiving of it.

When it comes to dealing with patients every healer has to be aware that each one is different and may need different approaches. Some respond only to the most physical levels; others may be more sensitive, they may already be experiencing certain phenomena and may want to learn and understand what is happening. Some who have been bereaved or are seriously ill may long for the comfort of spiritual perpetuation. Healing is not always about curing illness, often it is the attitude towards disease and death that has to alter. Many people come to healers as a last resort when all else has failed and they, especially, need love and peace, they need to feel safe and that there is some continuation beyond the body.

Sometimes healer and patient may not be compatible. Every healer has his own way and some may not be right for certain people. An example of this is a young woman who came to Philippa, having consulted a certain well-known healer. She was much disappointed because nothing had happened. She was experiencing intense pain, having

14

fallen and damaged her spine. Her doctors could only suggest a major operation with a 50 per cent chance of success and the possibility, if it failed, of being paralysed for life. After the first healing session the pain went. It returned again that night but, after more sessions, she learnt more or less to control it herself and was able thereafter to pursue a normal life. This is not to say that Philippa is a better healer than the well-known one; the point is that, for some reason, the young woman was able to relax with her whereas she could not before; she was able to calm herself so that healing could take place.

There is no doubt that miracles can, and sometimes do, happen. It is not really the task of this book to go into case histories, since it is concerned with how to heal people rather than people who have been healed.* Nevertheless, for interest we will cite briefly, in this introduction to the subject, the following cures which have been reported to the National Federation of Spiritual Healers.

Sarah, when she was born, was given little hope by the doctors. She was microcephalic, suffering from a rare disease which left her skull tiny and underdeveloped. Even if she lived a year it was thought she could never walk, talk or recognize her parents and it was advised that she be committed to a home. Her parents, however, were determined to keep her and when she was eight months old arranged for her to receive healing every week. After each session they noticed an improvement. Her head began to grow to a more normal shape, she seemed more alert to sound and to touch and, at fourteen months, she took her first steps. At the time of writing she is aged nine and making good progress at a special school, having just been awarded the title of 'Runner-up Horse Ranger of the Year'.

Audrey suffered a slipped disc which caused intense pain up her neck, across the shoulders and down the side of her head. After months of manipulation, heat treatment and traction she was no better and still experienced agonizing pain. One night she was sitting at home depressed and in great pain and her husband, who was becoming involved in

*See *The Power to Heal*, by David Harvey, Aquarian Press, 1983.

15

healing, came over and put his hands near her head. After a few minutes she experienced a pleasant warmth but dismissed the idea that anything could be done to ease her condition. The following morning, however, she could raise her head quite naturally and move it in a normal way, which hitherto had been impossible. Every restriction had disappeared and from that day she has experienced no further trouble.

Fourteen years ago Gail had a riding accident. Two bones were broken and her spine was slightly bent. Periodically, two or three discs would become displaced, causing considerable pain. Last December things went from bad to worse. With difficulty she made the journey to a leading back specialist three times but, although he had helped her previously, now, although he tried injections and manipulation, he declared the discs were too unstable and recommended surgery. In the New Year she had spiritual healing. After the first treatment she was free from pain and her spine straightened. Now, several sessions later, she is fully mobile and has gone from strength to strength.

Seven years ago Anthony had a serious motorcycle accident. During the succeeding years he experienced increasing pain and immobility in the lower spine, pelvis and left hip. The pain became so severe he was obliged to lie on the floor in order to dress himself and to watch television. Walking and gardening were quite impossible. He was told, meanwhile, that nothing could be done for him other than surgery. He had 'osteoarthrosis in the hip, scoliosis of the spine and spondylolisthesis of the vertebrae'. In this condition he received healing. That night he enjoyed the first painless night he had had in months and next morning he could dress himself without lying on the floor. At the time of writing he has been able to return to his yoga practice, to work in the garden and to walk for many miles each week. Although pain is still present it is usually mild by comparison.

Doray was working as a model when, aged thirty, she got cancer of the face. She had five major operations but it spread up the cheek and into the tear duct so that it was impossible for her to use her left eye. Into the bargain she had a bad back and was dangerously swollen with water – no diuretics

16

would work for her. Four years ago, in this condition, she was facing a sixth operation when she had one session of healing. That night she passed 8lbs of water and her back stopped hurting. Three nights later her eye cleared. From then on she got better and better and when she turned up on the appointed day for the operation she was told it was unnecessary. She was completely clear of cancer.

These are the miracle cures. But often the healing process is slow and almost imperceptible as the patient gradually changes in his attitudes and habits. Ultimately he has to take responsibility for his own health and it is sometimes necessary that he should participate actively in his cure, cleansing his system perhaps through diet and pursuing a programme of exercise. Sometimes a patient may not apparently be cured at all. He may not want to be well. He may be using his illness to attract the attention he feels he needs desperately. He may have no will to get better, no belief in anything. Although he goes to a healer, deep down in his heart the last thing he wants is to get better. An interesting experiment carried out among a group of students illustrates the effects of positive and negative attitudes. The group was given water and told they had just been given a tranquillizing draught. Some immediately said they felt calmer, but others said they felt ill and more anxious than ever. In other words there are some people who have negativity so deeply engrained that they will usually say they feel worse after treatment.

It is impossible for healing to take place without the chemistry of the body altering and the state of mind changing. There is no mystery about this. We can see from special monitors, equipped to measure brainwaves, that the minute a person relaxes a change of brainwave occurs. In other words, nothing can happen until the patient relaxes. If he is unable to relax it is unlikely that healing will take place. A friend of Lilla's took some ECG equipment into a prison in America and wired it up to some prisoners in order to demonstrate to them how their negativity affected their systems. Every time they felt resentful, angry or uneasy, every time they told lies, they could see this showing up on the monitor and whenever they felt better and relaxed they could see how this, too, produced a change in the rate of brainwave.

Often the developing healer will need to have his gift affirmed again and again. It is important for him to belong to a supportive group which will be helpful in building up his self-confidence. In order to be a good healer it is vital to work on oneself, to purify and go within in order to develop the necessary resolution and inner strength for dealing with other people's pain and distress. Above all it is important for the healer to understand what he is doing. For example, if he starts to heal before he is ready he may lose energy, feel disturbed or even provoke a heart attack. The point is that healing is not something with which to play around, especially if the healer himself has something wrong with his own body. Some, as they develop, experience very little, but some do feel changes and may experience certain phenomena. Some healers, as they grow in sensitivity, may experience symptoms, they may see colours, contact guides, have flashbacks to previous lives and so on. There are definite mechanics to the process of healing and definite tools and techniques. For some, perhaps, the idea of energy-centres, auras, guides, reincarnation and so on may seem irrelevant and weird. Indeed for such people these things probably are inconsiderable. They may heal on their own particular level without experiencing any changes in awareness or perception. But others do experience phenomena and this is why everything has to be taken into account and explained in order fully to be understood.

There is something else which should be understood in connection with the realization of psychic power and this brings the question of motive into perspective. Psychic power can lead an individual to enjoy great charismatic influence over others. If such a person is ambitious he may exploit this. If his motives are wrong, if, in other words, he is more interested in helping himself than in helping others, he can become a sort of psychic gangster who manipulates people for his own gain. We have only to look at the large following some of the modern gurus attract, at the programming that binds young people to some of the cults to see the truth of this. When we think of the Jonestown tragedy we can see

18

how dangerous this can be. Certain gurus are powerful healers but the thing to remember is that many heal people in order to demand their allegiance. To put it another way they practise their healing arts to establish a bond, a subconscious link with that person and then take him over. This is why it is important to be aware of these things and to go only to reputable healers who have no motive for healing other than a dedication to helping people.

It is worth saying here that when Philippa was first introduced to healing it was through just such a person.* The healing power came from her, she said, it was only through her that her disciples could heal. No one else had the authority. She was healing people, as were her disciples, as a preliminary to getting them into her power so that they would work for her (besides healing she liked her followers to do all kinds of chores including mending her sheets and pillowcases). Any doubts entertained, either about herself or her group, were proclaimed to be satanic. The truth is that she, and others like her, are exploiting people's fears rather than helping to overcome them. In her case many ended up not only frightened of her but also frightened to leave the group, since over and over again it was reiterated how dangerous it would be to do so.

This sort of megalomania is extreme. But it does sometimes happen that, in the course of his work, a healer becomes addicted to the idea of having power over others or, to put it another way, he develops spiritual pride. This usually happens when he uses mesmeric techniques or employs his mind over others. In any case it is likely that one who says bluntly: 'I am a healer: I can do this or that', is using other people as a kind of boost for himself. A true spiritual healer does his best to remove himself from the picture. He will never say that he heals people, only that healing happens through him, that he is simply acting as a channel.

It is important to clarify that spiritual healing is not being presented as an alternative to orthodox medicine but as a complement to it. No healer, or at least not one who is working within a recognized organization, would ever advise

*See *The Shortest Journey* by Philippa Pullar, Unwin Paperbacks, 1984.

patients to disregard doctors' recommendations or treatments. There is a vision of a new medicine in which doctors and healers work together in harmony. Healers could do much towards taking the pressure off GPs and alleviating strain on hospital services as well as reducing the annual bill for pain killers, tranquillizers and so on. Healers should work to aid doctors, never to supplant them – after all doctors, or many of them, should be healers themselves, that is to say, they should have healing qualities.

Organizations such as the National Federation of Spiritual Healers work to avoid charges of charlatanism by establishing an accepted standard and quality of practice and a code of conduct. Before healers are accepted for the referral list, which covers the whole country, their qualifications and performance are checked. The best way to find a healer is through recommendation but if this is not possible it is always wise to apply to a reputable organization. If a healer does not belong to an organization the patient has no redress, no body to whom he can complain.

1
Healing in Society: Past and Present

The art of spiritual healing is an ancient therapy which has been used throughout history. These days, in this so-called New Age, much of the traditional knowledge is being rediscovered and the power of healing is being taken more seriously. Increasingly, people are coming forward not only to be healed but to heal. There is a vision of a new medicine that is not so much revolutionary as evolutionary, in which doctors and healers work together.

In 1983, when Prince Charles opened Grove House, the new clinic for the Bristol Cancer Help Centre, which incorporates healing, vitamin and natural therapies, this seemed to be an official mark of approval for treatments which, hitherto, had been regarded by the establishment as fringe affairs. The way ahead appeared open.

Even so there is inclined to be an air of mystery hovering over the subject of spiritual healing, a hangover from the past, smacking of superstition and broomsticks. There are plenty of people who still feel nervous at the idea of receiving spiritual healing and probably the majority only consult a healer as a last resort when all else has failed. We need to know why this is so. We need to understand what spiritual healing really is and how it works so that all mysteries about this safe and practical therapy can be dispersed.

It is true that there are very few healers who are able to manifest the highest healing abilities of, say, Christ or Buddha — in fact, most people are not even aware that there *are* different levels of healing energy and that a healer's powers will depend on the level of vibration he can bring through. If we are seriously ill, if we have appendicitis, for example, most of us would rather go to hospital for an operation rather than turn to a healer. There is nothing wrong with this — we have to be practical and to use the appropriate means available to help and to heal ourselves. But it does raise the question: what has happened to the growth and development of our healing gifts? Why is it that, instead of being able to use our natural powers we have, to a large extent, lost them so that, for many of us, modern drugs with all their side-effects are part of daily life?

Beyond all doubt our technological achievements are considerable. They come as the result of fear: fear of pain, fear of death, fear of the unleashed powers of nature. Our scientific progress makes it possible to numb the body and the mind and to cut away the offending parts; it makes it possible to harness electricity and to gather energy from the elements. We have tried to safeguard our environment, but through our longing for security, through trying to make ourselves comfortable, we pollute ourselves and our surroundings and in consequence we suffer from disease and disorder. Most of us are unaware that it is possible to use our own bodies as transformers. We have so many possibilities for transmutation. We are here in the world with all the resources of nature at our disposal with which to create health. Instead, we produce disharmony. We destroy.

In order, first of all, to understand our present attitudes to healing we should see the historical facts that have gone towards shaping them. In the past every culture, every civilization, had its healing deities to whom were attributed miraculous powers of curing the sick. Next to gods, the healer-priests were most revered. They were the chosen few with access to the sacred source of life. They stood at the threshold of the physical world, able to reach beyond to those divine powers that could remove suffering and restore life.

In the ancient world education was available only in the temples. Knowledge was sacred and was revealed only to those proved to be mature enough to receive it and who could be relied upon not to exploit it for their own gain.

This was an inner circle into whose mysteries it was necessary to be initiated, for whom the penalty for breaking the rules and disclosing the secrets was death.

The general idea behind the training of neophytes was that of mind over matter. The aim was to learn to control energies, to harness, direct, channel and transform them, to raise the vibrations higher and higher in order to radiate them through the whole body. Neophytes had to work to purify the body, to focus the mind and unblock the energy. They worked for the means of gaining control over themselves first of all, thus ultimately demonstrating considerable power over others. In order to do this there were different exercises for discipline, awareness and quickening the energies. One way, for example, was to become so sensitive that you animated every nerve, enabling you to feel a colour or a sound right through the body; you *became* the vibration of that colour or sound.

The aim then was to contact the source of energy, or flux, and learn to control, channel, boost and transform it so as to be able to use it for whatever purpose it was required. Healing was only one of the ways by which the energy could be employed. Temple education was not specifically concerned with the healing arts – although some temples were known especially as centres of healing. The medical temple-schools of Egypt, for instance, were famous all through antiquity; their healer priests were dedicated individuals who spent the first part of their lives in acquiring the appropriate properties for their office.

The earliest known healer, or physician-priest, is Imhotep, said to have been one of the greatest of Egyptian sages. About his life and his work little information is available, but we can see the range of his knowledge from the impressive list of titles he bore: Grand Vizier, Chief Lector-Priest, Architect, Sage and Scribe, Astronomer and Magician-Physician at the court of King Zoser, Pharoah of III dynasty, 2980–2900 BC. We find in the Westcar Papyrus an allusion made to a wonderful feat of magic performed by the Chief Lector-Priest of King Zoser. He was, moreover, a master of poetry and composer of songs; his proverbs were handed down from one generation to the next; he produced works on medicine and architecture, some of which were still extant at the beginning of the Christian era. But it is really after his death that he seems to have performed most of his healings. His temple at Memphis was one of the most famous temple-schools and hospitals in Egypt while, such was the acclaim of Imhotep himself, that he was first promoted to a demi-god and then, later, in about 525 BC to a full deity. To his patients he would appear in dreams and visions, sometimes healing disorders with a mere glance.

In the ancient world much importance was attached to dreams and their interpretation. Incubation, or temple-sleep as it was sometimes known, or, in other words, dream-therapy, was a method of medicine generally used throughout antiquity and is still carried out today in at least one temple in India.* Details varied but the general principle was that the patients would come to the temple and after special cleansing rituals would be allotted special dream-cells prior to the sleep. The quality of this sleep was vital. The necessary trance-like state was sometimes induced by alcohol, by intoxicating fumes emitted from burning herbs or minerals, by datura or brews of acorn, barley, honey, blood and sacred herbs. The London-Leyden Papyrus informs us that isolation, silence and virgin-lamps – whatever they might be – were also means of getting the patient into a state of receptivity. The healing deity, with the appropriate remedies and suggestions, would then appear in a dream which could, if necessary, be explained the following day by the temple-priests and priestesses who were skilled in the arts of dream-interpretation.

This temple-medicine incorporated the laws of hypnosis and suggestion. By linking with the patient's subconscious mind his belief and expectation of cure could be programmed and the patterns reinforced by the priests and priestesses who, through their dream-interpretation, were able to introduce further suggestion to the effect that a cure had either

---

*At Mantralayam in Andhra Pradesh, the shrine of the saint Ragavendra. The story is that Ragavendra entered this tomb alive in August 1671 and here he will remain for 700 years praying for his disciples. Many pilgrims stay for several days and will not leave until the saint has appeared in their dreams, giving them guidance and restoring their health.

already taken place or very shortly would be doing so. It was on the whole a comforting process. The patient was supported by the god or goddess, the mother or father figure, who succoured him at his hour of need. It is worth pointing out that the principle of the therapy bears a relation to modern techniques of mind programming whereby the mind is introduced to the idea that illness can and will get better.

The temple priests and priestesses were not only skilled in dream interpretation but also in the knowledge of curative herbs and animal and mineral extracts. The Egyptians had a particularly impressive back-up pharmacopoeia for purifying the body and relieving symptoms and pain. This could be administered in pills, lotions, lozenges, ointments, gargles, salves, suppositories and enemas.

All ancient medicine, whether Egyptian, Greek, Chinese, Tibetan, African or North American Indian, shared the conviction, which is carried by traditional 'ethnic' methods today, that healing cannot be tackled on a physical level alone. It is not possible to separate the mind and the spirit from the physical body. The ancients understood the necessity of linking with the subconscious levels of the mind. They understood too how to use the natural earth energies in order to restore the body's natural healing forces.

Our ancient forefathers had a particular kind of vision of the universe. They considered the earth as a living body which was irrigated not only by aquatic streams and rivers but by currents of energy. These were a nervous system of telluric energies which could either well straight out of the ground like springs, affecting the surrounding area where they surfaced, or flow like rivers crossing each other at intervals. These junctions formed centres or points of power. In order to foster these and to channel the flux, stones and sacred burial places were erected at each junction point of cosmic and telluric energy. Later, temples, sanctuaries of healing and teaching, as well as dwelling-places for animals and people, were always built at these auspicious points where energies crossed. The famous oracles, for example, were situated by sacred springs, holy caves or trees. In ancient Greece the place where you stood as you took your prescribed medicine was considered to be of consequence. Certain spots were known to be more sacred, more powerful, than others and so were especially favoured.

The ancients, then, lived in balance with nature. They were aware of universal energy – of the energies of plants, trees and stones. They knew that certain places in the earth could amplify energies; stones, trees and buildings were placed especially to reinforce that amplification.

There is evidence that the Egyptians used the principles of amplification for cleansing and healing rituals prior to incubation. Daumas, who made detailed studies of the temple at Denderah, discovered a long corridor of concrete lined on both sides with what he called 'healing statues' whose sides were inscribed with sacred formulae and were provided with a drainage system which flowed away into cubicles of different sizes and heights. Daumas's conclusion was that water was poured down the statues so that it became blessed or, as people might say these days, 'vibrated'. In other words the water was made potent. From here it ran into cubicles, or bath-tubs, where the sick bathed, sat or dipped their ailing limbs. The whole building, he surmised, served as a kind of retiring house where the sick went for the therapeutic dream.

All ancient medicine also shared the conviction that disease was the work of demons, or evil spirits, which prowled unceasingly round the body perturbing it. Many traditions went on to say that each illness had its own demon which was of a particular hue. An essential part of the treatment lay in discovering the secret name of the demon and commanding it to come out. Incantations from the Papyrus Ebers are interesting and again bear a remarkable similarity to modern techniques. Here you visualized your medicine doing you good. 'Welcome remedy, welcome, which destroyest the trouble in this my heart and these my limbs. The magic of Horus is victorious in the remedy.' The principle lay in believing that the medicine would make you well and, once again, you invoked the support of the gods to help you.

So disease was due to possession by demons and one of

the most essential of healing arts was exorcism which, all through history, was used primarily for healing the sick. The aim was to expel the demon, thus releasing the patient from the fear and tension the disease was causing so that his own vital healing energies could flow. It is significant that the Egyptian hieroglyphic for fear is a goose, dead and trussed, demonstrating the paralysis of something winged which hitherto had been free. Another incantation from the Papyrus Ebers is indicative, both on account of the 'evil red thing' (which will be dealt with later), and the supplication that Isis 'might make free'. 'O Isis, great enchantress free me, release me from all evil red things, from the fever of the god, and the fever of the goddess, from death, and death from pain and the fear that comes over me.'

During the Graeco-Egyptian period the famous Imhotep gradually became fused with the Greek god of healing, Asklepios, to whom he bears a remarkable resemblance. Today Asklepios is held as the patron of all physicians, while his principle emblem, the snake-coiled rod, remains the specific symbol of medicine. Like Imhotep, Asklepios seems to have been a physician of some distinction. Like Imhotep, too, he was deified after death, becoming the centre of a great cult which spread all over the world, a characteristic feature of the worship being incubation. And, like Imhotep, it is mainly for his work after his death that Asklepios is best known; it is his dream healings that constitute his greatest claim to fame. Diseases vanished overnight, the sick woke free from illness. From the beginning Asklepios had, among his clientele, poets and philosophers to whom, apparently, he was not only the source of good health but also inspiration. His cures are documented by tablets in temples and he appears in a number of contemporary plays and works of literature. We read that in dream-apparitions he cut veins, operated, applied remedies and recommended treatment to be carried out at home. Sometimes his prescriptions included special diets and exercises, swimming in the sea or bathing in springs and rivers. By late antiquity there were hundreds of healing temples and shrines dedicated to the god of medicine who was supposed to appear nightly at all of them, but it was the cult centres of Pergamum, Epidaurus, Tricca and Cos, the great sanctuaries with their golden roofs, marble pavements, fine paintings and sculptures that were the most powerful and all who could, would make their pilgrimage to one of these.

Purity of the patient was considered vital. There must be the outer purity of ceremony and inner purity of heart. 'Pure must be he who enters the fragrant temple, purity means to think nothing but holy thoughts', reads one of the inscriptions over the doors. To ensure purity before the all-important temple sleep, the patient had to take certain preparatory steps. He had to cleanse himself – purification with water was important in Greek cults and sacred healing springs are to be found all over Asia Minor. There were other rituals which included staged processions and games, and sacrifice offered by priests in ceremonial robes of white and purple. Sacred lights were kindled, to be extinguished shortly before the god was due to make his nightly round. To help induce that essential trance-like sleep, rhythmic chanting, paeans and the recitation of poetry went on through the day, performed by regular choirs. At Pergamum, patients were required to pass down a dark tunnel pierced in the ceiling with shafts. The official tourist-guide explanation is that the priests above would call down suggestions and incantations to the patients in the dark below. It is possible, as at Delphi, that intoxicating fumes could have been introduced through the vents in the roof in order to change the consciousness of the patient.

The emblem of Asklepios, the serpent twining around the staff, is symbolic of the whole process of healing that went on in these sanctuaries. Here is the symbol of opposites: the serpent and the pole. One is alive, the other is dead; one is coiled, the other is upright. Together they show the union of opposites: they symbolize the healing process whereby man returns to the depths of his unconscious self and becomes healthy. Through integration of his whole self man achieves attunement and harmony.

So the serpent, together with the pole around which it twined, represented total fusion, it was a symbol of man's most holy goal. All through antiquity snakes were held as sacred and this is still true today in many parts of India. The snake was believed to be the embodiment of the god himself and it symbolized the rejuvenation he brought about. Every Asklepion had its sacred serpents, along with other ritualistic animals, particularly dogs, sparrows, geese and cocks. As soon as a new temple or shrine was established a sacred serpent or two would be dispatched thither by carriage or ship. Testimonies on the temple-tablets record incidents of serpents appearing, even in broad daylight, licking wounds and restoring sight. Ladies in their dream-cells would be joined by serpents which, according to the tablets, would lie down beside them and cure them of their barrenness. Indeed, licking by sacred serpents and dogs was a well-known household remedy and was considered to be highly efficacious.

The ancients were always fond of having tame snakes around to guard their houses and their temples. The figure of a serpent appears as a personal or house-protecting amulet all through Egyptian history. On one level it could be said that keeping snakes was quite practical. It was a good way to stop anybody from stealing treasures in a temple, or anywhere else. But there are subtler reasons than this for regarding the snake as holy, as an integral part of temple life.

Like the initiate the snake grows for the duration of its life, every year shedding its old skin and starting again with a new one. This continual process of growth and rejuvenation is symbolic of the initiate, of the primal instincts stirring and demanding to be transformed. It stands for the word 'initiation', itself – the new beginning. The human being because of his appendages, his tensions and fears, often causes his vitality to stick somewhere. One of the main lessons of the temple exercises was letting things flow. Snakes were often used by initiates who were working to achieve a free stream of energy running through their bodies. They would observe how the snake's energy courses smoothly, without restriction. They would hold them, move their hands down them, feeling how the release system worked. They would allow a snake to wind itself round their limbs and watch the change in energy.

In some of the sacred dances the hand and the arm emulate

the actions of the cobra. Such dances were exercises in feeling, in sensing, in becoming the snake, in becoming fused with it in one constant flow of energy. They were exercises in awareness and mind control. Sometimes neophytes had to learn to use that particular type of energy in order to control the snakes themselves. Serpents featured variously in some of the initiatory rites. One of the tests was to try your mesmeric powers: to see how frightened you became and to see who controlled what. You might be enclosed in a pit or a cave with poisonous snakes, together perhaps with large cats, which you would have to control mentally. If your powers of mesmerism were inadequate and you were unable to project your mind strongly enough the animals would kill you and you would have failed the test.

Snakes, then, were sacred creatures which were carefully tended in the temples and were integral to the oracle, the mystery cults and the arts of healing. The fact that the serpent was especially sacred to Asklepios, who was supposed to appear in this form, may have contributed to the Christian enmity towards him and made it particularly easy to see the pagan deity as an incarnation of the devil.

To the Church, trying to establish itself as a political institution, the cult of Asklepios presented a serious threat. By the beginning of the Christian era, worship of the god of medicine had spread through the world of antiquity. By the second century AD, although other cults had lost much of their grip, the authority of the Asklepions was at its height. Worship of Asklepios was a powerful living force. 'Thousands excited over him as if over a saviour', complained Eusebius. The basic reason for disquiet lay in the fact that Jesus, in appearing as a physician and healer, resembled Asklepios more than any other pagan divinity. Indeed there was an astonishing similarity. Both were sons of God and of mortal women – Asklepios was believed to be the son of Apollo and of a lady called Coronus – both had come into the world to heal the sick and raise the dead. (Legend has it that Asklepios was struck down by Zeus because he went about during his life raising the dead; through this he was violating the laws of the universe so Zeus struck him with a thunderbolt.) To the followers of the Greek god, Christ appeared to be just another Asklepios while, to the Church, Asklepios was the devil, its strongest enemy, drawing men away from the true saviour. 'He is the arch-demon', wrote Tertullian. And this designation held; several centuries later Bishop Alcuin was referring to Asklepios as 'the false Christ'. Gradually, though, as the Christian Church established itself, the popular appeal of Asklepios declined. The great sanctuary of Pergamum, with its golden roofs, was destroyed by an earthquake between the years 258 and 260, was not rebuilt and the stones of the temples were taken to build Christian churches. The holy places became quarries for the Christians.

In the beginning the early Christians had themselves been powerful healers – it is said that even St Peter's shadow had healing powers. Jesus' last words, when he appeared after the Resurrection and described the signs and wonders that would manifest in all who believed in him, are famous: 'They shall lay hands on the sick and they shall recover.' Healing, though, was only one of the gifts of the spirit that could manifest. Others were the casting out of devils, prophecy, the working of miracles, the speaking in tongues and the interpretation of tongues. These were all diversities of gifts out of the same spirit. 'We have amongst us' Tertullian wrote,*

> a sister whose lot it has been favoured with gifts of revelation, which she experiences in the Spirit by ecstatic vision. . . . She converses with angels and sometimes even with the Lord; she both sees and hears mysterious communications; some men's hearts she discerns, and she obtains directions for healing for such as need them. Whether it be in the reading of the scriptures, or in the chanting of the psalms, or in the preaching of sermons, or in the offering up of prayers, in all these religious services matter and opportunity are afforded her in seeing visions.

Divine possession, in other words possession of the human body by the god or goddess, was well known throughout

*Quoted in *A New Eusebius* edited by J. Stevenson, SPCK, London, 1957.

antiquity. The oracle, for example, was consulted on all matters from national importance to personal health. The god or goddess would possess the priestess and speak through her entranced utterances. In Israel there was a long tradition of inspired prophecy, the prophet in an ecstatic state believed himself to be the mouthpiece of God, the vessel of the divine, who spoke through him. To the early Christians possession by the Holy Spirit and the gifts that ensued was deemed a most valuable experience and was actively sought – indeed, divine possession, direct experience, played an important role in the public relations of the early Church, impressing pagans and making converts. There is the famous occasion on the day of the Pentecost when everyone started speaking in tongues. The apostles were sitting in a room when there came the sound from heaven as of mighty rushing wind and what seemed to be tongues of fire appeared. The apostles were all filled with the Holy Spirit and began speaking in tongues. The din was such that other people thought they were drunk and the situation had to be explained by Peter.

In those days speaking in tongues seems to have been quite common among the early Christians. Paul's first letter to the Corinthians suggests that those first assemblies were singularly noisy with the congregation being visited by the Holy Spirit, some beginning to prophesy while, simultaneously, others spoke out loudly in tongues which nobody could understand. Paul was obliged to lecture the Corinthians on the need for greater order and good sense. Supposing outsiders, unbelievers, entered and witnessed the scene, he remonstrated, would they not think everyone was mad? There should be less noise and more interpretation; all things should be done decently and in order.

It is interesting that the picture presented of these early assemblies could scarcely be closer to today's revivalist type of worship in which possession by the spirit of God creates and reinforces faith among the people. In the 'bible belt' of the United States, revival meetings and chapel services engender tremendous religious enthusiasm. Among the gifts manifested through possession by the Holy Spirit is believed to be the power to handle snakes: 'They shall take up serpents.' This has been taken literally by some American sects. The psychiatrist, Doctor William Sargant, witnessed and described some of the snake-handling ceremonies.* Rattle and other poisonous snakes are gathered in the mountains and kept in boxes. When it is seen that the Holy Spirit has descended on the meeting and possessed the congregation the elders open the boxes and hand round the snakes which the congregation take up and whirl about. Sometimes they get bitten, sometimes not. Doctor Sargant observed that the congregation, having danced and sung themselves into a state of trance, displayed all the signs of being hypnotized. The ceremonies seem highly therapeutic. Many of the snake handlers that Sargant saw were poor people who lived in squalid conditions and were on the whole downtrodden and exploited. For one day in the week they could work themselves into states of emotional excitement, rid themselves of the previous week's tensions and frustrations and start again with a clean slate.

Back in the early centuries of the Christian era manifestation of the spirit and realization of gifts among the congregation began to constitute as much of a threat to the Church's authority as worship of Asklepios. The last thing the Church wanted was the sort of chaos that was felt would come to pass if everyone went round displaying powers. It was not so much the power of God that was exercising the Church; rather, it was the political predominance it wanted for itself. To be functional the Church needed to establish a theological system which was outward looking and allowed no personal interpretation or emanatory experience on the part of the individual, no personal knowledge of the supernatural.

The idea was that, since no members of later generations would have the access to Christ that the Apostles had enjoyed, every Christian believer should look for knowledge to the established Church, to its gospels and its bishops. It waged a vigorous campaign against any Christian group whose belief threatened to be subversive to clerical authority. The Gnostics, for example, the men who knew, were expounders of the ancient wisdom. They had inherited the

*See *The Mind Possessed* by William Sargant, Heinemann, London, 1973.

33

unwritten law, the oral tradition which was only made known to those who were instructed in the mysteries. They advocated that all who reached Gnosis transcended the Church and the authority of its hierarchy. Gnosis revolved around intuitive reflective processes of self-exploration and the Gnostic texts are remarkably oriental in their pursuit of personal experience and personal union with the divine – pursuits which not only undermined the bishops' authority, but also made them redundant. Altogether the Gnostics were viewed as highly undesirable and volumes of vituperation were levelled against them, accusing them of sorcery, magic and carnal goings on.

Self-knowledge was undesirable and so were the ancient practices of using natural energies. Various passages in the Bible reveal that some of the prophets and Israelite leaders were versed in the ancient knowledge. They knew how to exert the energy of stones and amplify it by sacrifice – all through antiquity young animals, birds and even people had been sacrificed so that the released energy could be applied. Just to take one example: we find Moses (Exodus 24:4) rising early and building an altar under the hill, together with twelve pillars, according to the twelve tribes of Israel, and dedicating burnt offerings and making sacrifice of oxen to the Lord. The blood was then sprinkled over the altar and over the people gathered together.

Now the Church forbade all ceremonies involving the use of stones and trees and all visits to the oracle. Any form of psychic exercise or gift, including that of healing, was absolutely discouraged. All divination, prognosis and astrology was forbidden while belief in reincarnation was anathema.*

For reasons of politics the Church effectively confiscated all the levels that lie between the devil and the angels (and, as we shall see, recently they have tried to do away with the devil and the angels as well). It might be helpful to imagine these levels as corresponding to the colour spectrum; in other words the Church shut the door on the whole range of

*See *To the Light* by Lilla Bek and Philippa Pullar, Unwin Paperbacks, London, 1985.

34

colour, leaving only black and white: the lowest and the highest. This made transmutation or transformation, which had been the whole essence of temple training, extremely difficult since all techniques using intuitive awareness or energies of the sun, the moon, of stones, animals and trees – all the energies of nature – were forbidden. In other words, the working areas had been closed up.

On one level, aside from political motives, you could say that the Church was trying to provide a teaching that took people as far away from the primitive side as possible; it was trying to quicken a sense of the highest and most beautiful. In essence, you could say, the whole of the church service was an amplification, all the ingredients, the mass, the holy relics, the candles, the incense, the rituals were designed to boost energy and raise the consciousness. But the consciousness had to be raised unconsciously. There was no explanation, little instruction, apart from being told to lead a good life and love the neighbours. The Church was trying to convey a way of channelling energy into the body directly through the highest archetypes, through white light. This is a difficult thing to do because, in order to link with white light successfully, we have to be able to accelerate our vibrations to the necessary rate and if we do not have the necessary power ourselves we will need those techniques of amplification which were suppressed by the Church.

Aside again from political motives the Church's attitude towards healing was largely influenced by its view on sickness. Sickness, the official line had it, was the result of sin and God alone had the authority to heal. Sickness was the result of sin and healing was a matter for forgiveness alone. From AD 314, beginning with the Synod of Ancyra, a number of decrees were issued over the years variously forbidding the practice of healing. Any attempt to heal was seen as evidence of paganism or devilish inspiration, or both, and healing became associated with sorcery, smacking of magic and paganism.

All over Europe and into Britain, Christianity spread and shrines and churches were erected on the sites of ancient temples. Legions of Christian saints, many of whom had

35

been branded as sorcerers and executed by the Romans,* occupied the sites of sacred springs and groves, and spells and incantations were uttered in the name of Jesus Christ. Where possible the old customs were bent and authorized in the name of Christ, but where this was impossible practices were forbidden and that which had hitherto been held as sacred was denounced as profane. The legend of St Patrick expelling the snakes is interesting here. The ancient ring forts of Ireland, surrounded by stone circles, are believed by some to be fortresses of the Sidhe, the prime magicians of Ireland. They were fortresses above and sacred tombs below, used for rites of fertility and divination, in which it is thought the oracular serpents were kept.† (W. Stukely in his works on Avebury and Stonehenge also submits that these megaliths were connected with serpent worship.) Serpents, being sacred and integral to ancient tradition, would naturally be viewed as evil; there could be no possibility of including them under the Christian umbrella so they were deposed.

Nevertheless, in spite of Christian advances, the old knowledge, the old ways continued. People would resort to traditional practices. Over the years the bishops would be obliged to issue warnings. 'Before all things I declare and testify to you that you shall observe none of the impious customs of the pagans,' warned Eligius in the sixth century,

> neither sorcerers, nor diviners, nor soothsayers, nor must you presume for any cause nor for any sickness to consult or inquire of them. Let none presume to hanging amulets on the neck of man or beast even though they contain the words of the scripture. For they are fraught not with the remedy of Christ, but the poison of the Devil. But let he who is sick trust only in the mercy of God and receive the sacrament of the Body, Blood and Christ and according to the apostles the prayer of Faith shall save the sick and the Lord shall raise him up.

---

*It is ironic that the greatest sanction which the Romans could use against dissidents to the regime was to brand them as magicians and sorcerers, for which they were punished by death. Hundreds of early Christians were thus branded and executed, many, in time, to be beatified by the Church.
†See *The White Goddess* by Robert Graves, Faber & Faber, 1961.

'It is not allowed for any Christian man to fetch his health from any stone, nor from any tree', added Bishop Aelfric.

There were, however, ways round the prohibition. Intercession with the saints was permissible. Any cure affected by the saints was evidence of a miracle, of God's generosity. Bishop Aelfric, who was obliged to scold a sick man whom, in spite of his warnings, had been trying to fetch his health through forbidden practices, recommends that he should seek his health at holy relics instead. Bede tells us how Bishop Germanus of Auxerre came to Britain in the fifth century with a casket containing relics of the saints hung round his neck. Filled with the Holy Ghost he performed two healings with his casket, applying it first to a blind girl's eyes which apparently emptied of darkness and filled with light, and then to a boy's withered limb which filled and the muscles regained their power marvellously.

This, basically, is the situation as it stands today. The Church has always feared the attainment of psychic powers and those who deal in the supernatural. During the Middle Ages any such activity was denounced as heresy and punished by death. In condemning sorcery and witchcraft the Inquisition was actually concerned in stamping out direct mystical, direct religious experience, and its inevitable associations. The Witchcraft Act, which carried with it the death penalty, was repealed only thirty-five years ago in 1951. Up until then any lay healer was liable to be arrested.

In these days much traditional knowledge is being rediscovered. For this there are various reasons. Over the past twenty years there has been a great wave of interest in anything occult. Ironically, the Church, doing its best to keep up with the technological age, continues to play down all supernatural elements, feeling that they have no place in modern life. It is true that, within the Anglican Church, there are a number of healing groups together with a Christian parapsychological movement, the Churches Fellowship for Psychical and Spiritual Studies (CFPSS)* which issues a quarterly journal, *The Christian Parapsychologist*. But these are

*The equivalent group in the USA is the Spiritual Frontiers Fellowship.

sophisticated, fringe activities. What we are talking about is the main body of teaching and traditional opinion. Meanwhile, hundreds of people, reacting to the materialistic twentieth century, search for religious experience which is more likely to be pursued through Eastern traditions, hallucinogenic drugs and the occult than through the orthodox Christian Church.

Our mission in this era has been to develop the intellectual, mental, scientific, technological aspect, generating thereby the stamp of the individual. Through our genius we can now gather energy from the elements, we can travel to the moon, split the atom and alter the genetic code. Never, it seems, have we possessed such extraordinary powers, yet our intelligence is threatening to destroy us. On the one hand we have the extraordinary developments of science; on the other, the degradation it has created which threatens our civilization. In reality we have created an absurd world. In the name of efficiency the individual has been turned into a consumer, an object to be used for consuming, yet, due to technology, machinery is replacing him and he does not have the salary to perform his function and to pay for his consumption.

In another field there is growing dissatisfaction with the limitations and shortcomings of modern allopathic medicine. We have conquered TB, smallpox, plague and leprosy, yet something always turns up instead. Cancer, heart disease, multiple sclerosis and AIDS are the terminal diseases of the twentieth century against which science fails to make any substantial impact.

Thalidomide has shown that the side-effect of drugs can be out of all proportion to the benefits. Melville and Johnson* calculated that more people are killed each year by prescribed drugs than by accidents on the roads. Iatrogenic disease – disease that is caused by drugs – is an enormous and rapidly growing medical problem. Stress is so prevalent today that the anti-stress industry is one of the few boom businesses in the economy, along with alcohol and tobacco. Every doctor's waiting-room is crowded with patients suffering from the

*See *Cured to Death*, by Arabella Melville and Colin Johnson, Secker & Warburg, London, 1982.

strains of the twentieth century and the easiest way is to prescribe sedatives, tranquillizers and sleeping pills. Here is one of the areas where lay-healers could be of considerable use to doctors and the overburdened Health Service. They have the time to listen to people and to care for them.

The astronaut, Captain Edgar Mitchell (who participated in the third trip to the moon) has drawn a parallel between the ancient therapy of acupuncture and spiritual healing.* Westerners, he said, had practised acupuncture for some time, but it took a trip by two scientists, Arthur Galston, a biologist, and Ethan Signer, a physicist, to travel to Vietnam and China and bring back the story. Eventually, after other scientists and finally President Nixon had also visited the East, acupuncture burst like a bombshell upon the United States. What happened to acupuncture, he believes, will happen to spiritual healing.

Not to make use of the available resources is as impractical as dismissing the very real benefits that allopathic medicine has to offer. We have overdeveloped the male aspect of our natures. The pendulum has swung too far in the direction of the masculine and the intellectual and we have reached a point where we need the intuitive, the female side of wisdom, to regain the balance and bring the opposed aspects together in mutual stability.

*See 'New Developments in Personal Awareness' by Edgar Mitchell, *The Dimensions of Healing*, Academy of Parapsychology and Medicine, Los Altos, California, 1972.

2
The Evolution of Energies

It is essential for a healer to comprehend the nature of energy. He must understand how energy moves in the universe and how it functions within himself. A healer's body is his instrument, his tool for channelling and releasing energies. Without knowledge of how this works, he is like a carpenter who, without knowing either his materials or his tools, tries to build a cabinet. The famous words inscribed over the temple at Delphi and Eleusis endorse this: 'Man know thyself.' To know yourself was the key subject of temple curriculum.

First, we need to discuss the nature of energy itself. We have to say that 'energy' is an inadequate word: it has, in these days, such an industrial ring to it. Our language is unsatisfactory when discussing these subtle esoteric ideas. If we could write in Sanskrit or Chinese we would have more possibilities with which to define what we mean. With Sanskrit, for example, *prana* is transformed from *retas*, the lowest sexual energy, to ever finer expressions until, ultimately, there is *ojas*, the most luminous kind of energy. It may be that the reason our language is so wanting in such terms is that, up until now, the supernatural has more or less been ignored. The levels between the devil and the angels, the centres of energy within the body, were not recognized so there was no need for a vocabulary with which to describe them. These days, however, modern physicists are coming up with discoveries that affirm the visions of the ancients. Fritjof Capra, for one,* has shown clearly how the insights of new physics mesh closely with those of the mystics and it is significant that, in order to convey this information, it is

*See *The Tao of Physics* by Fritjof Capra, Wildwood House, London, 1975.

sometimes necessary for scientists to invent new words and new terms.

In any event we know from physics that all matter is a whirling mass of movement containing no isolated lumps. It is continuous dancing, vibratory motion whose rhythmic patterns are determined by molecular, atomic and nuclear structures. The atom itself is no more than an area of space wherein electrical forces establish the nature of the nucleus and its associated electrons. Each atom is a field of energy possessing positive, negative and neutral charges capable of producing electric and magnetic forces.

When Lilla first began to see these energies and to observe how they moved, she found it difficult to describe what she was perceiving and almost impossible to explain these things in tangible terms. She felt there must be something on earth that would be able to give her some clue, some idea of continuity. So she turned to nature to discover if she could distinguish any of the shapes she was seeing. It was the moving waters of the sea that first gave her insight. Here, in the different movements, the waves, the eddies, the whirl-pools, were clues. By looking at the waves rolling on the beach, or at the centre of a whirlpool sucking in the water, at the rise and fall of tides, we can see patterns which repeat themselves in exact proportion through nature: in the spiral of a shell, in the rings of a tree trunk, the petals of a daisy, the fronds of a fern unfolding towards the light.

All energy, all the forces of the universe, are movements which emanate from one source, one point, the centre of all consciousness. They radiate out in all directions, travelling through space in rhythmic vibration in the form of waves. The point of distance from crest to crest is known as the wave-length, the rate of vibration is known as the frequency. The movement of life is a rhythmic pulsation, an expansion and contraction, which is reflected in the changing cycles of the year, in spring, summer, autumn and winter, in the waxing and waning of the moon, in the heart-beat and the breath. The flower, the tree, the crystal reflect the order of the world and express divine harmony. Light, colour and sound manifest the rhythm of life. Everything which is perceived is a succession of impacts. Night and day, the changing seasons, these are all a rhythmic succession of changing movements which link every existing thing. Each individual possesses a biological clock which is attuned to this universal movement. The earth, the moon, the planets, revolve round the sun. Our galaxy moves in reference to other galaxies. The universe expands at a given moment and will contract. A perfect correspondence links our heart to our respiration. Everything in nature, every person on earth has a beat and, if the rhythm is too fast or too slow, illness ensues.

In the temples the initiated priest raised the demarcation line between the tangible and the intangible, united the eternal with the ephemeral. There is only one world, its two aspects are visible and invisible. Its energies change from subtle to dense, from chaos to order, and back again from order to chaos. Thus the invisible is linked with the visible world. In Indian mythology the all-embracing serpent is often seen as a symbol of creation, the bridge between the material and the immaterial. It may imply a constricting power which embraces or limits. For, without limitation, there can be no direction, no inside and outside, no here or there, no foundation on which to build. Before there can be a concentration of energy, the means of producing an effect, there has to be a limit to space. The serpent emerges from the egg as a line from a point, when the head and tail meet it makes a circle; linear expansion is thus limited and becomes measurable. The unlimited expansive power of creation is embraced and thereby the content becomes knowledgeable.

The universe is silent and colourless and it is only through impact on our senses that the splendour of the world is generated. The movement of life manifests as innumerable possibilities in vibrations or oscillations. Here is a creative force of countless different wave-lengths and frequencies but, so long as we remain in the body with its limited sensory abilities, we can perceive only a few of them. Our organs transmit the vibrations to our consciousness and, according to the sensations we receive, we may perceive matter, sound, heat, taste, smell, thought, ideas and light.

For practical purposes we can say that these wave-lengths manifest in seven rays of vibrating currents which appear as near as possible to the colours of the spectrum. Every type of creation, from the celestial bodies down to the amoeba, is the effect of various forms of these rays all issuing from the one original beam of light. Every form of creation has the possibility of reflecting through it and manifesting that original beam of light – we can call it what we like – God or the universal consciousness. Everything that exists carries this point, this spark of divinity, within itself. This spark exists in all things and in all creatures. When we can recognize this spark of divinity permeating the universe we can recognize the essential oneness, the essential unity in all things. If we are unable to see the soul, the spirit, the spark, in people we will be locked forever into the physical dimension. The spark is eternal and with it the idea of age vanishes.

If we took a section through the spinal column of a vertebrate, we could see that the energies most permeated with this vital spark are in the centre; the further out from the centre, the denser, the more material they become. We would see the fine substance of the bone marrow at the centre which carries the creative force, protected by the dense structure of the bone. This is equally obvious in the stem of a plant or the trunk of a tree. In the centre, fed by the tree's innermost energy, the circles of vitality radiate out and are protected by the hard bark. This life force is present in every creature and manifests in countless variations on every level. Every form reveals only so much of that original spark, that original beam of light, as it can experience consciously.

Perhaps the most important point in the idea of evolution is awareness or consciousness: the raising, whatever the species, to ever higher levels of awareness, the unfolding towards the light, the progression towards ultimate perfection. Animals, vegetables, minerals and humans depend on the degree of consciousness and mobility their genus has attained. The mineral, at the lowest level of consciousness, manifests itself through contraction: a cooling off and a hardening. The plant level of consciousness is the vegetative force which gives life to matter and manifests itself unconsciously in the search for, the absorption and assimilation of food. Animals have three forces, material, vegetative and animal: they have bodies, they seek out food, they absorb and assimilate it and are conscious on an animal level, enjoying emotions, instincts, urges, feelings, desires, sympathy and antipathy. Each of these groups is progressively one octave removed from the rest, only man has the power to manifest several degrees of consciousness. The average man stands one octave higher than the animal. He has a body, he seeks out food, he absorbs and assimilates it, has emotions, drives, desires, sympathy and antipathy and, above this, he is conscious on a mental level, he has intellect and ability to think.

In the temples neophytes were trained to gather energy, channel, transform and release it. They worked to accelerate their vibratory rates and strengthen their bodies so that, ultimately, they could consciously experience the highest intuitive levels and transmit them through radiation. In fact, the human body is geared automatically to raising the vibrations ever higher. We all long to feel happy, to feel 'high', yet most of us are unaware of how to sustain this state of well-being and the only way that energy can be experienced rising up and releasing beyond the body is in sexual orgasm. It is interesting that, in the cruder forms of American revivalist celebration, as Dr Sargant observed, the worshippers are encouraged to 'come through' to Jesus, to have an orgasm: if an orgasm occurs it is taken to be a sign of the Holy Ghost.

Different schools, different disciplines, civilizations, mystery cults and religions have methods of instruction for controlling and channelling energies. The Chinese, Hindu and Tibetan are among those who talk about centres or points of energy. They suggest specific exercises of breathing and chanting for focusing the mind and stretching the body in order to direct and channel the flux. Such religions do not discourage the development of psychic powers. The Tibetans, for example, have always believed the attainment of psychic powers to be well within the capacity of man and beneficial if properly used. All, however, are agreed that such manifestations are not an end in themselves but should be part of spiritual growth only, otherwise they will be a distraction from the true path.

The Christian religion is one of the most inexplicit of schools and, as we have seen, has abolished the practical working areas, dealing only with the highest levels which are difficult to accomplish without instruction. This makes transmutation extremely difficult. 'Lift up your hearts', is one of the more specific prayers: in other words, here is an instruction to raise your vibrations to God, to the highest levels of consciousness.

Yet transmutation, or transformation, is a necessary ingredient of psychic survival and growth. Our job as a human being is to be a transformer of energy, to be able to create high-level radiations. The well-known healer Bruce MacManaway has a useful analogy. 'Imagine the main electricity cable,' he says, 'with a tremendously high voltage flowing through it that somehow needs to be transformed; in order for you to use it for your hairdryer or kettle the voltage has to be stepped down. The human being, and especially the healer, does something of that sort.' Through our systems we absorb different types of energy. At the lowest level we transform food into vitality for the brain and body consciousness and with the lungs we transform air or prana into food for the spirit. We must never limit the idea of healing just to the laying on of hands or taking away sickness; it is the growth of everything we touch upon.

Matter is changed by our conscious state. Every time we touch anything we change it, so that if we are in a bad mood and touch something we will have a lowering effect. We are here to transmute everything, everything we buy, everything we inherit. Lilla once knew a young man who worked hard at his emanations and became a marvellous transformer. Once he washed her clothes and ironed them for her and it was sheer ecstasy to wear them.

So how does the system operate? Within the body the field of energy is divided into different levels which correspond to frequencies of the colour spectrum. Seven vital centres are situated down the spine from the top of the head to the sacrum and are known as *chakras*. These seven main chakras are attached to the spine by cords which have roots and the general appearance is that of flowers. Knowledge of this chakra system is essential because it is through this that the

45

healing process operates. The chakras control the organs of the physical body, together with the neuro-endocrinal system. Besides the seven major chakras, smaller ones are situated in the shoulders, knees, ears, hands and feet, while thousands of tiny points of energy are situated all over the surface of the skin. All these chakras, no matter whether large or small, are transforming stations, they are like power points which transform high energies from other planes down to vibratory rates which we are able to use on the physical body. Unless we are receptive to a vibration it will pass through us without our being able to make use of it – this is true of all levels; no matter how good an idea, how wise the words of a teacher, they are going to make no impact unless we are ready and willing to receive them. Without these transformers, energies from the higher planes would simply enter the body in the form of physical energy and there would be no capacity for thought or higher values. We would be unable to exhibit emotions and ideas.

At the core of every chakra is a black and a white hole. Here are the two polarities, the two complementary opposites that are contained within us all, the two sides of nature which are eternally at conflict one with the other. Here is the ability to go to heaven and the ability to go to hell, the possibility for good and evil, the masculine plus aspect and the feminine minus principle – which are so beautifully represented in the Yin-Yang symbol. We cannot have a positive potential without its correspondent negative counterpart. Even in the minutest structures we can find these plus and minus principles. The black hole gathers energy by bringing in strong forces from the cosmos and passes them into the white hole which gives them out again. Thus one sucks in energy, drawing in nourishment as a plant draws in water; the other releases it like a fountain. Goethe describes this beautifully: 'We all have certain electric and magnetic forces within us,' he wrote, 'and ourselves exercise an attractive and repelling force according as we come into touch with something like or unlike.'*

*See *Eckermann's Conversations with Goethe*, translated by R. O. Moon, London, 1951.

When the chakras are about to open the energy increases until a compelling centrifugal action forms an aperture. The stable points of the chakra, though forced apart, still maintain an attraction towards one another. When the flow decreases the points should resume their original pattern but, if any centre opens too soon or too emphatically, the power will surge through the centre and if the points are weak and do not for any reason possess a firm pattern of attraction then the centre may sometimes remain open which is unhealthy. With some people the chakras can open easily, with others they stick. Some people in an emergency seem unable to help anyone, they are unable to cope with anything, while others speed up in emergencies and are active and competent.

The chakras, then, are like cups of energy which, when open, seem like hundreds of chalices, large, medium, small and tiny, all open and full of light. Good or bad energies may be attracted depending on the state of the chakra; the subsequent interaction propels the chakra into a circular motion. Different chakras have slightly diverse ways of accumulating and maintaining energies. Those at the top should be quicker and more subtle. This, however, is not always so; coarse vibrations can and do appear in all centres.

Our transforming or healing potential can only start when we are able to open all the centres. In the temples neophytes would learn to open and close each centre at will and to balance them. This is important. If we are unable to control ourselves and we do not have the stability to cope with the forces we are channelling they will be useless and probably destructive as well. It is only through being able to open to the higher energies that a healer is really capable of healing. But in order for us, human beings, to be able to function on the higher levels and to reach our full potential we have to create a resonance field capable of receiving the higher vibratory rates – and to achieve this the ancients used techniques of amplification.

Energies change constantly and in the course of evolution the human body has developed so that, on the whole, our centres are larger than those of our forefathers. To put it another way the size of our chakras depends on the stage of our evolution. It was in fact easier for the ancients to control their energies effectively. Not only was the potential of the earth's radiations stronger, not only did the temples provide a protective environment, but the energy centres of human beings were smaller and therefore easier to control. Clearly it is not useful to have large centres if they cannot be restrained. To be endowed with too much energy, to be over-charged, is as useless as having too little. The constructive use of small centres can be more potent than the inability to control larger ones – however, it is difficult to heal people who have larger energies or faster vibratory rates than our own.

Actually, our own universe bears little resemblance to that of antiquity. Although the earth's energies have risen to a higher level, much of the environment is polluted and people find themselves with centres that are difficult to synchronize. In these days we have also a strong ego-consciousness which strengthens from generation to generation and becomes more and more difficult to deal with. Long ago people were much more collectively conscious, much more group oriented. You could say they were more of a group soul. If the father was a cobbler, the son became a cobbler also. There was a tradition of handing down knowledge from father to son, master to apprentice. Now we have become individual to such an extent that usually children are completely against anything their parents want them to do. We should have reached the stage in our evolution where we are able to control our egos, yet our personalities, having learnt how to survive and preserve themselves, have grown in their self-consciousness.

We have now to take the step from self to cosmic consciousness. We have to become like the snake, one of the most successful and adaptable of species, which is able to establish itself in any area (apart from the polar regions and – because of St Patrick – Ireland). These days we have no external temple environment; our mission is to establish that security within us so we can take it with us wherever we go, to any place in the world we happen to be.

The Bodies of Man

Man is composed of a number of interpenetrating vehicles, the densest and most familiar of these being the physical body, a highly complicated machine, without which it would be impossible to gain certain experiences on earth. This body must be looked after in an intelligent way for, if we abuse it, we suffer. Never must we forget that we are spirits inhabiting a material body which is vital for our growth and development. Earth is a good school, but it is not the spirit's true environment. The spirit has to be protected. We can think of man's various bodies as coating for the soul; these bodies are layered, rather like the skin of an onion. When the physical body is linked and in harmony with the other bodies, when it is provided with correct nourishment and its zones of elimination are working efficiently, it should maintain a state of well-being and radiance.

Disease manifests when the physical body is cut off and unable to oscillate rhythmically with the other bodies; when vitality is impaired and poisons build up. One of the reasons why so many people need healing is that they move their bodies badly; the way they move their hands, their limbs, never allows the system to clear. Most people, for example, never stretch their limbs fully.

Human physiology is dependent on harmonious, rhythmic attunement. Health is the expression of this order. We do not find the sun rising at six one morning and eight the next, the planets darting about in a haphazard way, or the ocean tides going wrong. Yet we, humans, indiscriminately break all the laws of nature, then wonder why we are ill.

The physical body consists of various conduits and organs which are governed in the spinal column and the brain by the seven main chakras, each of which aligns to a major endocrine gland. These chakra-endocrine pairs are major energy modifiers which should work in synchronization with each other to process the electro-magnetic vibrations of certain wave-lengths. Many diseases arise as a result of excessive or defective hormonal secretions released from various glands into the blood or lymph. Stress, for example, will produce too much cortisone and the immune system will go down.

So to understand the healing process we should understand something of the neuro-endocrinal system. We can think of hormones as crystals circulating through the body carrying the vibratory rhythms which are picked up by the glands and broadcast in terms of required function. The principle is similar to the radio sets which were made with crystals to pick up and interpret the radio-waves. Hormones are messengers: they tell the body what to do. Governed by the chakras, the neuro-endocrinal system works to establish a harmonious internal environment. It controls the circulatory, respiratory, digestive, lymphatic, nervous, muscular, skeletal, reproductive and excretory systems. We can see now how the under- or over-charging of one, or of several, chakras will cause the vital energy to become blocked and injurious hormones to be released which will disrupt the function of organs and glands.

The strength of hormonal secretions is shown here by an illustration from an American biology text-book. Epinephrine, the secretion from the adrenals, is so potent it can still be detected in a dilution of one part in 300 million. In other words, if one ounce of this substance were to be so diluted with water the solution would fill nine miles of petrol lorries: nine miles of petrol lorries; 268 lorries to the mile; each lorry holding 2000 gallons and you could still detect epinephrine in that dilution. Another researcher has isolated a hormone from the pituitary which is so powerful that 560 miles of such lorries would be required to reduce one ounce to an undetectable point. With our mind, with our thoughts, with the thought of resentment, joy or compassion, an immediate response goes through the autonomic and then through the endocrine system and the most imaginably minute secretion can affect every cell.

The nervous system is constantly at work. It is not unlike the administrative offices of a government, being arranged in networks and ganglia which are strung up and down each side of the spine. Alternatively, it is sometimes likened to the tree of life: the sap, the energy, rises up through the spine or the trunk and travels out through the branches. Here is the major source of energy to the body. From the spine the energy travels through the whole body and beyond. Although it influences all organs the first to be affected is the glandular system through the release of hormones. It is not difficult to see how healing techniques applied along the sides of the spine will affect the whole of the body and the brain.

The etheric body is an exact replica of the physical: a field of energy surrounding and supporting the physical body which is composed of interchanging lines of force. The reason we can still feel an amputated limb is that, although the physical has been removed, the etheric is still there maintaining a balance. Where an intersection occurs we find a chakra; where several intersections meet we have a minor chakra and where the major junctions arise we have the main chakras. Here is the same principle as the universal network of energies; often the telluric energies have exactly the same structure as our etheric bodies.

In relation to the physical and etheric bodies it is significant to cite the researches of Dr Giuseppe Calligaris,* professor of neurology and psychology. He discovered on the surface of the human skin a complex system of lines forming every kind of geometrical shape. The structure of these lines followed a general tendency in nature, the same patterns that are to be found in honeycombs, crystals, leaf structures and so on. Where the lines crossed they formed contact points, or what he calls 'plaques'. He estimated there must be millions of plaques on the human skin which are all interconnected, each with a fixed relationship to a specific point in the brain and a particular inner organ in the body (these do not correspond exactly with the points of acupuncture). Plaques, he claims, are doors through which vital radiations may stream in and out. Each respective radiation has a door through which it enters from outside space and a door through which it leaves. The stimulation of these plaques has the effect of opening the door so that the corresponding rays can stream through. A mechanism is released which gives direct access to the subconscious; the normal sensory

*See *Precursore di Una nuova Era* by Giancarlo Tarozzi and Maria Pia Fiorentino, Casa Editrice MEB, Turin, 1975.

perceptions are bypassed and the person in question can go beyond the limitations normally experienced with the consciousness. The subconscious is lifted to the level of the consciousness and the person receives extrasensory perceptions beyond his usual realms. Through stimulation of various plaques Dr Calligaris's subjects were able to see spirits and ghosts, enjoy clairvoyant and telepathic skills, read thoughts, detect lies and observe the landscape of stars, together with the vegetation and inhabitants of other worlds outside the normal time-span. The skin, he concluded, works like a magic mirror where everything is contained. But only a fragment of these mirror-images ever rise up out of the subconscious to reach the consciousness. There has to be a filter system otherwise the consciousness would be overwhelmed by a chaotic abundance of information. The complete universe can be merged on the skin of the human body. This bears out the view of the Chinese who see man mirrored in nature and only understand him as they understand nature.

The astral or desire body uses the same system as the etheric body but functions on a faster vibratory rate and penetrates each chakra with its own essence. This astral or, as it is sometimes called, desire body, is one that causes most of our problems. Desire, ambition and emotion play an enormous part in our lives. Like everything else they have two complementary aspects, positive and negative. It is through desiring to change, desiring to grow and to develop, that we will do so. But if we continually desire pleasure this will be destructive, and can become obsessive. Instead of just wanting something we can become obsessed with it so that the need will take us over. It will control us rather than us controlling it. In these days we are bombarded with advertisements. Constantly we are urged to enjoy ourselves sexually, to eat, drink and be merry, to have more and more possessions. The result is that we become unbalanced.

When someone becomes emotionally disturbed the astral body does not function well and this will affect both the physical and the etheric. When all these are unbalanced we will radiate bad energies. Then everywhere we walk, everything we touch will emanate negativity which in turn will affect people who are vulnerable and sensitive and make them ill.

The mental body is not just a small compartment situated somewhere in the head, nor does it have to be encased in any shape. All the other bodies have the mental body inter-penetrating and spreading through them, extending well beyond the physical body. Indeed the mental body is capable of going whither it is projected – across the world, into the solar system and to other galaxies. But its potency and effect will depend upon the strength of projection, which depends ultimately on the strength of mind. The mind is the reality, the other bodies are merely instruments to be used by the mind and are dependent on its state. What the mind is the body must be. The energy flows through us and the form it takes will be determined by our thoughts.

Our whole circulation is affected by the mental body. Mental blocks restrict the circulation of the etheric and blockages in the etheric are similar to clots of blood in the physical and can cause all kinds of illness. If the mental world is perturbed and we are frightened this will act on the heart, which will act on the blood circulation, which will alter the energy-fields. A simple anxiety will change the whole process. Incorrect thinking causes disharmony to every cell and organ. Correct thinking is healing.

Let us briefly take the idea of belief. It has been proved by orthodox medicine that, in 40 per cent of cases, placebos will cure the disease. What does this mean? When you believe a medicine is active and will do you good (as in the case of the Egyptian incantations) your thought process, instead of having a blocking effect, will enable your dynamic energy to take over and you will heal. Thought is responsible for the whole complicated alchemical process of the body and will affect the glands – as will the things we say. Everything has to be performed mentally before it can be expressed physically. All matter is really materialized thought.

The mental body is subdivided into several levels, a bit like a staircase climbing ever higher. For simplification we can divide it here into three main sections: the conscious level, which controls the physical body and *all* its functions, the subconscious levels which link into the collective consciousness and the highest intuitive levels, which we can call the superconscious, with which we will deal later.

We can compare the vehicles of man to a complicated electric network. We know that with electrical wiring if there is a breakdown somewhere a high voltage will appear in other places. This is precisely what happens with the human body. For the mind and spirit to be able to work in the physical body there have to be laws. The spiritual force is far too strong to operate without a system of voltages. If an organ is disturbed the normal resistance will break down with the result that a higher voltage will appear in other points and will affect the flow of the circulatory system. Every action has its effect. If we clench our hands full of anger and tension we are likely to affect the thyroid. Irritation can cause problems with the kidneys and the inability to release resentment will affect the excretory zones. The liver also suffers from anger, so do the eyes. It is important to remember that every emotion has a vibration and if, instead of being able to release negativity through the excretory zones, we send it up the body and express it through the mouth it can have an unfortunate effect. If we have to release our frustration and emotion by saying how dreadful a person is we are not really releasing, not really emptying it out of our system, we are just reinforcing it and producing a lot of dark energies that will ruin the circulation, unbalance the thyroid and thymus and affect the pituitary and pineal.

The Aura

Surrounding the physical body is a protective electro-magnetic field which can be observed by seers and which is composed of radiations formed by all the bodies of man. This aura should be felt and understood by all healers since it is one of their main tools for cleansing, transformation and protection. A good therapist needs a large aura and to be able to use it efficiently he should use all the techniques at his disposal. Again and again he will be told that being with him is soothing; that it is good to be in his presence.

Children and animals will want to be with him, nature will respond to him. A big aura is the equivalent of someone standing with his arms open ready to receive you.

The aura appears as a fountain of energy and when radiating competently has a definite and regular shape. If it bulges in some places and seems lacking in others it demonstrates that its owner is also out of shape. Most people have no idea whether their radiations extend more in front than behind, whether they are stronger in the feet than the head. No-one is identical and the size of an individual aura will depend upon its owner; the healthier a person the more regular his energy-field will be. In any case our emanations change constantly according to the seasons, fluctuations in the weather and our moods. There are times during our monthly, weekly and daily cycles when they will pick up strength and radiate better than at others, times when they will be more resilient, times when they shrink and times when they open.

Our auras are absorbers, soaking up vibrations from everything around, the sun, moon, animals, plants, stones and people. They develop as the consciousness develops. As with chakras, it is easier to live with a medium-sized aura than to live with a large one. A large aura is difficult to control since it can dissolve people's thoughts. The larger the aura the more thoughts it can dissolve; this may lead its owner to feeling depleted. The weaker a person the more he is susceptible to other people's energies and the more he will take on their projections. So we can say that a strong aura will influence another. Let us imagine that a healer meets an overactive person. His aura should have an overall calming and stabilizing effect, he should be able to pacify his patient with his emanations; alternatively, if he meets someone lethargic he should be able to give him a charge of energy.

Above all, the healer's aura must be still. The healer should have an inner calm, an inner beauty. There can never be a real change in humanity while we, humans, continue to look only at the physical body. Sometimes people seem really ugly yet they have beautiful auric spaces, beautiful emanations and, of course, the opposite also holds true. We have to be aware of our auric space, we have to make it beautiful and to know that, through its radiations, it is capable of transmuting negativity.

The Second Nervous System

It is not generally realized, or at least not here in the West, that all animals and all men possess a second system which passes along beside the familiar central nervous system and which has been known in the East for hundreds of years. When looking at evolution we can see how the success of a species depends on its ability to sense danger. In the beginning the full-time occupation was survival: reproduction and the assimilation and excretion of food. Survival is a primordial instinct in animals and men. One of the functions of the autonomic nervous system is to make its owner sensitive to and aware of danger. We will, for example, instinctively jump away from the heat of a burning object and so avoid hurting ourselves.

As all forms of life were evolving two nervous systems were required. One, the autonomic system, reacted to close stimuli, the other, second, system allowed the man or the animal to sense danger at some distance away — hurricanes, for example, earthquakes, the approach of predators. Nowadays there are still people who are able to foresee disasters, earthquakes and pending deaths and accidents. Wild animals retain their sensitivity to environment, indeed their survival depends upon their innate ability to sense the approach of predators and the location of food supplies. Early man would never have lasted had he not enjoyed the same aptitude, sensing the approach of strangers or wild animals from great distances away. Furthermore, he knew instinctively which plants were good to eat and which were not, by being drawn to them or repulsed.

These two systems are common to all sentient beings, but in animals they function only automatically and are still geared to survival. Humans, however, can exercise this circuit in order to develop the mind and raise the consciousness. In order to evolve we have to rise above the levels of survival and grow towards illumination. Indeed, this progression is a natural law which can be seen reflected through nature. If we take an example from the kingdom of plants, we find the rose, whose bud unfolds towards the light, drawing the sap up from the earth and transforming it to a subtle perfume. The ancients knew that, by coordinating the highest mental levels through the full use of the circuit, the faculty for higher perception could be developed. When the system is operating correctly the whole of the skin surface will send signals to the inner system; like feelers it can gather information from the environment. We have seen that every element, every substance, every body, has special radiations or vibrations and we know that the human being is capable of sensing whatever is in his environment. One of the aims of martial arts is to discover and develop an awareness of outer space so that the student will know spontaneously when anyone approaches.

Early man, then, for reasons of survival, concentrated on his outer space. Though his internal chakras were smaller than our own his surface chakras were larger and more active. Indeed he was highly tuned to his skin surface and it was natural for him to pick up immediately if something was wrong. It was not until he had settled down into villages and eventually towns and cities and was living in comparative security, no longer requiring his system for safeguarding his outer space, that he began to develop his mental and intellectual powers. We have seen that, within the security of temples, neophytes were able to focus their attention on their inner space. The temple dances had a dual purpose; they sought an awareness of what was happening both inside and outside the body.

These days our space is almost entirely alien to us. Most people are unaware either of their auras or their external space. Most of us, in other words, have become so introspective that we are quite insensitive to our environment.

3

The Levels of Healing

It is not generally understood that the power of healing manifests in different rays which correspond directly to the rainbow. Although we could say that healing is really a case of accelerating the body's own capacity to repair, build and maintain itself and that in reality, no one heals another person, he only helps his patient to heal himself by giving him a charge of energy. Nevertheless, what we are talking about here is the quality and degree of light the healer can bring into his body. The quality of his powers will depend on the vibratory rates he is able to channel.

Ultimately we should be able to reach the point where we can use all the rays. It is through being a rainbow and manifesting all the colours that we, as human beings, can evolve. So it is essential that any potential healer should develop his colour range.

When thinking of the various healing rays it is helpful to imagine them as gears which change upwards, always faster and higher. So we have the base, the bottom chakra which governs the excretory zones, corresponding to red, the abdomen to orange, the solar plexus to yellow, the heart to green, the throat to blue, the forehead to indigo and the highest to purple. To give an idea of this let us suppose that we have a patient who is deficient in sexual drive and vitality and who has arthritis. It is likely that he will need an injection of red energy. Some people want yellow, they lack the security of practical logic, the structure of the analytical and geometrical aspects of the left brain; they are unbalanced in that they are too intuitive. Others may be saturated in the yellow intellectual ray and require the blue intuitive radiation.

At the basic level nearly everyone can project some sort of healing energy, even if it is just through helping a person sit and rub a leg. You could say that by your very presence the person will be encouraged to massage their limb more readily. So on a very fundamental level you can help a person get energy into their body by some form of physical manipulation. Actually some people are very physically oriented and unless they swallow something, or are massaged and manipulated in some way, they will not believe that anything is happening.

When dealing with the physical body it is often best to be practical. It is difficult, for example, to find a healer these days who is good at setting bones; neither are healers, on the whole, good at dentistry or extracting bunions and callouses. Healers can get rid of many things, they can replenish and realign anything that is necessary but, unless the patient ultimately takes responsibility for himself, he will forever be leaning on the healer or therapist. Some people may need to change their diet, they may want herbs to purify an organ, they may require to have their bodies realigned. If someone's neck is out of place that individual will continue to have headaches; if he carries on wearing clothes that are too tight pain may recur in various parts of his body. If neither patient nor healer are aware that the circulation is being restricted, the patient will keep coming back for healing because he is continuing to do the wrong things. This applies equally if he is sitting, standing or walking in the wrong way.

On another level, it is possible to heal with the will or imagination. We can will people to get better. This can be helpful. Beyond doubt many individuals have weak minds and someone with a strong will encouraging them, saying: 'Come on, I'm sure you can do it', may give them a boost so that they can reinforce their own mind. But really a healer should not interfere. His job is to act as a channel: he should offer his energy, his heart and his skills without willing, wanting or imagining results.

Before going further it would be helpful to understand the principles of magic. Magic is an understanding of the hidden laws of life. Black and white magic are two complementary aspects of one force and they can work only if they are channelled. Thus we are the tools of black or white magic according to our awareness. To bend the forces of nature to our own will for our own good makes us black magicians; to bend them in the light of evolution, in order to help humanity and nature, constitutes white magic. We, human beings, are entrusted with the earth. We are here to embellish rather than exploit it. It could be argued that defying the laws of nature and violating them, manipulating the genetic code, creating the atom bomb, are all feats of black magic.

The traditional black magician uses the lower chakras and channels the reproductive and earth energies. Rituals and ceremonies, involving dancing and sexual celebration, provide the necessary boost to his energies by pumping them up and stimulating the adrenal glands. It is exciting stuff and addictive. Often adepts feel strong and powerful and will be able to heal quite successfully. Gradually it becomes necessary for this type of magician to use ever wilder rituals and ceremonies involving stones, sacrifice and often alcohol, to raise the energies. In effect he is a collector of energy rather than a transformer. He can collect energy and transfer it, or he can in the early stages, but he is unable to transform it since he does not employ the higher chakras. Thus any healing he gives will not be real since nothing will change. It will be unlikely that he can deal with diseases requiring the higher vibratory rates. There is nothing really wrong with borrowing things providing we give them back. Black magicians, however, live off borrowed energy without returning it. They are parasites. But it is impossible to borrow all the time without something rebounding. And there is another point. If we approach any source of power and bend it with motives of our own gain, the energy will eventually cause our disintegration.

We have always heard that we can ask the devil for power and he will give it to us but, in the end, he will destroy us. Goethe's Faust is such a tale. Life is movement: a rhythmic expansion and contraction. Through the practice of black magic the energy circuits become overcharged and the physical body manifests disturbances. The movement of life is disrupted. As pressure continues to gather the hormonal secretions produce poisons, bodies become heavier and

60

heavier and the person in question starts to emanate negative vibrations. Generally, the heaviness manifests as a palpable force which in its turn attracts evil. As the coarse particles accumulate the etheric grows darker until the physical body degenerates. We can see this clearly demonstrated through modern techniques of photography. It is possible nowadays to reproduce diseased and healthy cells and observe that, while the aura of a vital organism has a lovely even contour, that of an unhealthy cancerous cell appears heavy and shaggy. There is nothing wrong with the force that gathers energy, just as there is nothing wrong with the slower vibratory rates, providing they are correctly used. Because something is intense does not mean that it is bad. Indeed, without the force of gravity we would be unable to exist on this planet. We have to live here on this globe, to be practical and down to earth; without the forces of gravity we would be unearthed, unable to function in a practical way. The force of gravity and the black hole will destroy us only if there is something wrong; then we will disintegrate until we can gather ourselves together again and go towards the light.

Red Ray

This is the dynamic, sexual and reproductive radiation, the heaviest and slowest vibratory rate in the spectrum. Many people who are ill need this basic hot energy – chronic diseases nearly always require heating up. When patients say they experience heat going into the body it is this quality of power going into the spine. These warm energies have to be used for charging a patient so that his vitality can be rekindled, but we must realize that the pleasant warmth they engender can, for some people, lead to sensual reactions. We have all encountered people who are oriented to sex and who have earthy vibrations. In any case a healer who projects these warm waves easily will be able to help those who are suffering from arthritis, rheumatism, lumbago and sciatica, any stiffening of the muscles and joints, any systems that are generally sluggish.

This vibration draws poisons, builds up red corpuscles,

stimulates arteries, sluggish menstrual discharge and the autonomic nervous system. If vitality is lacking, a simple remedy is to wear red underclothes and if there is any trouble with the blood it is good to drink carrot, beetroot and red grape juice.

Orange Ray

This is an active ray, a mixture of intellectual and reproductive energy. On this ray healing works through action: helping a person to exercise, for example, cooking the right food and so on.

All early systems of medicine involved some form of activity in order to create the indispensable energy. Most traditional shamanistic practices involve dancing in a circle to the regular beat of drums, sometimes with the aid of alcohol or drugs. Their aim is the therapeutic release of emotions. Dr Sargant witnessed many healing dances in Africa and Brazil and noticed that most of the ceremonies included periodic breathing or chanting, together with rhythmic stamping movements. The dances would culminate successfully with the patients falling entranced to the ground, crying, writhing, in a state of collapse, releasing thereby all tension, anger, fear and hostility. These trance-dances, Dr Sargant observed, effectively broke up the patterns of behaviour and emotion that had gone before and in this context Sargant makes an interesting observation: the new youth culture of the West, which is based on frenzied dancing to the pounding repetitious beat of music and drums, has helped to create the permissive society and bring down a whole structure of belief and convention.

No real shaman, witch-doctor or medicine-man uses only dance, drums and chanting. These, on the whole, serve only to make the patient receptive. Many use the ritual of sweat-lodges whose functions include the release of poisons and negative emotions. Most are experts in herbs and diets. Many will suck a wound or affected part and are seen to vomit out the poison. Some may charge up their hands by rubbing them vigorously together and make long sweeping passes down the body without touching. Some make the same movements but use feathers. Most will question the patient in the first place to see if his attitude is positive. Why does he want to feel better? What will he do when he is? Is there anything he would like to improve or to change?

Another who has made an extensive study of the methods used by shamans is the Mexican, José Silva. He has been to Brazil and the Philippines observing witch-doctors and psychic surgeons and has devised a commercial healing course using techniques based on their ritualistic practices. He includes the rapid passes, the long sweeping movements made down the body, the hands being rubbed together vigorously beforehand, at the same time as drawing a deep breath. These passes, he claims, excite the molecular particles in the body.

The orange ray increases oxygen, helps lungs and menstrual cramp, encourages interests and activities, releases gas, draws boils, brings abscesses to a head, depresses the parathyroid and stimulates the thyroid and a mother's milk.

Yellow Ray

This is the ray of intelligence or intellect. It is possible to imagine a patient getting better and to heal him in this way. But we must realize the level of our visualization. If we imagine someone's insides are like a plumbing system and that we are clearing out a dirty drain this is really visualization on the orange level. It is better, if we are going to use visualization, to bring in the higher colours, to introduce nature or put the patient into a fountain of golden or white radiations. In other words it is better simply to put the patient in the light and leave it at that. Most children, however, do seem to need the active ray for their visualization exercises to be successful. Imaginative techniques seem to work best with them when the images are aggressive – knights fighting dragons perhaps, sharks gobbling up little fishes.

So it is possible to heal with the mind through imagination. There is also hypnotism. Many good hypnotists get to the root of the problem but sometimes a hypnotist can convince a person that he will have no more pain: the pain will vanish all right, but the cause of the suffering will still be there. In other words a tumour can continue to grow painlessly until eventually it kills the person. There is the story of a woman who went to a hypnotist wanting to give up smoking. This she was able to do sure enough, but her system immediately turned to something else since there was a basic need which had not been dealt with. She started to eat enormous quantities of sweets instead; when that was stopped by the hypnotist she began sucking her fingers, then biting her nails and, eventually, she became an alcoholic.

Beyond doubt there are people from all walks of life with magnetic personalities who can mesmerize human beings and make them do almost anything they want. Their success is due to their large energies. Often they are overwhelming, attractive individuals who, when they meet a person, will give him their attention completely – and this in itself is very seductive. Often they have the power to inspire their followers with great enthusiasm – some of the charismatic healers move large audiences, hundreds of people at a time. Sometimes such healers do inspire individuals to find their own path, but some of these mesmeric healers have ulterior motives for giving healing. Many enjoy the power it gives them. Many give healing because they themselves are insecure and long to be wanted and appreciated, long to be liked. Healing satisfies this urge and makes them feel that they can achieve something. Generally the patients become deeply attached, mesmerized in other words, and will return to these healers again and again.

It might be helpful here to look briefly at Franz Anton Mesmer himself, who gave his name to mesmerism and who graduated in medicine in Vienna in 1764. Around 1766 he came up with the phrase 'animal magnetism'. This was a force, he believed, that existed everywhere in nature, was concentrated in magnets and issued from the hands and the nervous system of the physician or mesmerist. His treatments were famous. He used a large wooden tub in which were placed a layer of glass and a number of bottles containing iron filings. Protruding from the tub were jointed iron rods which were attached to the ailing limbs of the patients who would be arranged round the tub in several rows and connected to each other, either by holding hands or by cords which were passed round their bodies. No efforts were spared to make the scene as impressive and dramatic as possible and to give the effect that mysterious powers were at work. The lights were dim, the hall thickly curtained to maintain silence, music played while Mesmer dressed in exotic clothes prowled round in the background carrying an iron wand with which he touched the afflicted parts of his patients. Sometimes he stared at them, sometimes he seated himself opposite, foot against foot, knee against knee and rubbed the affected part. Sometimes he made magnetic passes or stroked them. This might continue for hours. Effects of the treatment varied – some felt nothing, some thought insects were crawling over them, some coughed and spat, some fell into convulsions. This last was called the crisis and was considered highly beneficial; it seems similar to the state engendered by the trance-dances: involuntary jerking movements of limbs and body, rolling eyes, nervous excitement and tension, leading eventually to a state of collapse and highly increased suggestibility terminating in a dreamy sleep.

A pupil of Mesmer's and a retired physician, the Marquis de Puységur, experimented with Mesmer's methods and decided that it was the somnabulistic or trance state induced by the mesmerists which was the therapeutic instrument. Gradually, the technique emerged that today we know as hypnotism.

Mesmerism is really a kind of theatrical act and often requires a lot of dressing up and setting the scene. Through these mesmeric levels you are really trying to put a person into a trance state in which you can persuade him that everything you are going to do will make him well. To psychic vision this sort of energy, which can either be projected mentally or by rapid passes, appears from the eyes, the hands and sometimes the pores of the skin, as a shower of tiny arrows, or even minute snakes, which dart from the mesmerist. Some mesmerists, or hypnotists, can and do use the higher levels, some use only these lower mesmeric ranges and project this shower of energy over their patients. This may have a tingling effect or the patient may feel that he is wrapped in a cocoon. Indeed there are some people who long to be enveloped in another person's emanations. It makes them feel that they do not need to take responsibility.

So, as Mesmer discovered, there is an electro-magnetic force that emanates from us and which we can channel to help others. But the spiritual healer can go higher: he can go through and gather energy from the cosmos. He can go through to the highest energy-fields within himself, to his higher self and, in so doing, he will awaken his patient who will be touched and illuminated. He can raise another's consciousness in order to create possibilities, rather than taking him over. The mesmeric healer who uses his own energy is not offering his patient the opportunity of trans-formation and he will make him want to return again and again. Healing should be a spiritual experience. The spiritual healer can transform a patient by touching him, sometimes by sitting with him and hardly touching him at all. He transforms the patient so that his own higher self can come through. He will make his patient feel that he cares, but he will not in any way hold on to him. His patient can go away and feel completely free. We could, for the argument, say that Christ had charisma. Yet always he directed the power and the attention back to God, back to 'my father in heaven'. He never kept it for himself. He was, moreover, austere and his healings were without the showmanship that so many charismatic healers employ – so many need to rely on a theatrical performance to reinforce their hypnotic powers. It is, of course, possible, as we have already seen, to use the yellow ray for healing without any form of hypnotism, which is only one aspect.

Clearly no patient can be kept well if at some deep level he, himself, wants to be ill rather than healthy. We know that ancient systems of medicine operated on the assumption that when a person believed in something he changed. This is often demonstrated in psychic surgery. It is frequently not so much the surgeon or even the operation, as the trust, the belief of the patient in the ability of the healer or surgeon to make him well that does the trick. Certainly many psychic surgeons have an impressive ritual. Those of the Philippines are well known and draw bus-loads of foreigners. All kinds of matter from cysts and tumours to eyeballs are seen to be extracted. Blood often flows freely and the extricated tissue is clearly visible. The principle here is that, with an outward function, it is often possible to produce an inner change. No doubt some of these effects are produced by sleight of hand; it is animal tissue and blood rather than that of the patient that is brandished about. Nevertheless, the point is the power of suggestion, the influence of mind over matter, just as with incubation or temple-sleep. If a patient is not receptive to a change of vibration, such manifestations, whether experienced in dreams or day-time consciousness, can sometimes help him to change his mind. If he grasps the idea that something is being done and believes that the offending part has been cut out, his body and mind may accept that healing is taking place and allow the flow of vitality to unblock and the balance of energies to be restored.

There is a story of Lyall Watson's illustrating this. Lyall Watson was travelling in the Amazon with three Brazilians when one suddenly developed a fever due to an inflamed abscess under a wisdom tooth. Luckily a famous healer lived nearby to whom they repaired. The preliminary consultation was not concerned with symptoms but explored the patient's entire life and all the circumstances leading up to the illness. The healer's diagnosis concluded that the patient had been invaded by evil spirits. For treatment the healer lifted out the tooth as easily as though it had been lying there loose and, making the patient sit back with his mouth open, he massaged the swollen glands in his throat. The healer then sat opposite and began to sing softly. After a few minutes a trickle of blood began to flow out of the corner of his patient's mouth, followed by an ordered column of black ants. This continued until there were a hundred or more ants pouring out of the patient's mouth, down his neck, along his arm and on to the log where he sat. He and everyone else watched the column move across the clearing, into the grass and away; and everyone roared with laughter. It turned out that the local word for pain was the same as that used to describe ants. In an elaborate pun the pain had walked out. It was a symbol that the mind could easily deal with.

This vibration can help mental illness. It reinforces self-confidence and courage, helps assimilation, stimulates lymphatic glands, liver, gall bladder, eyes and ears, aids elimination of calcium and loosens deposits of lime that cause arthritis. It is helpful, if you feel intellectually debilitated, to tune into yellow flowers and yellow jewels. Lemon juice will help to loosen congestion and mucous.

Green Ray

This ray incorporates wisdom and intuition. As soon as we reach this vibration we begin to deal with the higher vibratory rates. One of the points about this radiation is that it may have no obvious reaction. The patient may experience nothing in the way of heat or coolness and may doubt that he has received any healing at all. Healing through the heart involves the powers of love and nature. One of the most healing things is to grow vegetables, then to cook them with great love and to feed that love to people. This is a beautiful living meditation. If a healer's heart is not really concerned with love of human beings and nature he will be using the left-brain hemisphere and his energies may not be balanced. Nature and animals are great balancers and in themselves are great healers but we have to approach them with love rather than with intellect. If a healer has no love he will be unable to channel this ray and it will be almost impossible for him to help people with cancer. Indeed, without the balancing force of the higher energies and the use of the right-brain hemisphere it is possible that his treatment could actually cause problems rather than relieving the illness. It cannot be reiterated too often that many illnesses cannot respond if the healer is not able to channel these higher vibrations since it will be almost impossible to bring about any change.

This ray stimulates the pituitary and raises the vibrations; it restores balance and builds cells, it is good for open sores, cuts, bruises and scars. It dissolves blood clots and heals infections. When healing on this ray we can use the hands to massage in aromatic oils and we can use herbal remedies.

Blue Ray

Through this radiation the whole atmosphere becomes calmer, it creates a protective capsule, a womb in which people feel happy and safe. All healers in the course of their spiritual progress must acquire a specific amount of this ray.

This level also deals with sound. Christ healed with his voice – so did many of the ancient healers as indeed do many shamans and medicine-men in these days. They command the disease, or the devil that caused it, to leave the patient. Lyall Watson's healer sang to the spirit to make it come out.

The voice, like everything else, can operate on different levels. We can think of sergeant majors and all like them who use their voices to give loud orders; university lecturers and teachers whose job it is to put ideas together and project them; we can think of actors, opera singers, politicians, priests and psychiatrists, all of whom exercise their voices in different ways, on different levels, in order to achieve results. The healer works to open his throat chakra so that he can bring through information from the intuitive levels to help his patient.

Repetitive chanting, like repetitive movement, forms patterns which help to change the brainwave. In the beginning, sacred music was often played for inducing trances and was associated with the sound of nature, ripples in the water, grass waving in the wind. The Druids became entranced by listening to the wind in the sacred oak groves. If you chant mantras, the roof of the mouth, which is an important and often neglected part of the anatomy, is changed in shape. The sound goes up and rolls round the dome of the mouth, hitting the pineal and pituitary glands. So, by chanting mantras and sacred names over and over again, you can put yourself into hypnotic states wherein you can reach deep subconscious levels. This, however, should only be done under supervision. After a little while all sorts of negative things can surface which sometimes need professional help. Singing in the bath is marvellously cleansing. Water helps to purify the etheric and the sound will dissolve any negativity that has been washed out and is hanging about in the atmosphere. But on no account should mantras be chanted in the bath. It would not be safe to chant oneself into a hypnotic trance while sitting in the bath.

This ray is good for sleep. It helps fevers, infections, inflammations, mental depression, irritation, itches and burns — coconut oil and Vitamin E are also excellent physical remedies for these last three.

Indigo Ray

This is a calming, pacifying, passive ray which affects the right side of the brain. It is especially important when treating neurotic people and those who are suffering from upheavals in consciousness. Acting as a sedative it is essential for any kind of nervous disturbance. It is the ray of intuition and the key to the intuitive levels.

We have seen that modern physicists are coming up, in the course of their researches, with conclusions and visions similar to those which mystics have been bringing through for centuries. The gap between scientific and intuitive knowledge would seem to be narrowing. Yet conflict remains still between those who deal with the left brain and those who deal with the right.

Perhaps the most dangerous aspect to the intuitive levels of the superconscious is the fear and superstition they sometimes engender. All through history people who do not, or cannot, practise their intuitive faculties have been afraid of those who do, and have persecuted them. Actually the only way we can conquer superstition is by using logic, or the left brain. There is really no such thing as bad luck. When a person is strong and healthy and his vitality is functioning correctly he will be able to transmute anything. Bad luck will only work if we allow it. Let us take an example: suppose that you walk under a ladder believing it to be unlucky. Because you are superstitious your energy levels will go down. You go round the corner and trip over something and you put this down to the fact that you walked under the ladder. There is nothing wrong with the ladder. It is you, yourself, that has caused the accident to happen. What is wrong lies inside you.

Long ago potions and amulets were common means of averting bad luck. There were amulets against the evil eye, amulets for this, amulets for that and there were love potions. Nowadays potions and amulets are coming back. People make quite a living selling them. You can see any amount of advertisements in magazines. If you buy a special necklace you will get this, if you buy an elixir you will get that. This is exploiting fear and is the last thing we need. What we do require is a clear sense of intuition so that we can know the truth for ourselves; know how to help people deal with their fear rather than exploit it, know also the important difference which lies between superstition and the symbols or signs which appear at certain times in our lives in dreams, or as coincidences (Jung calls it synchronicity), to make us see our paths better or to warn us of danger.

Intuition is a tool which needs to be backed by study and contemplation and which must be constantly observed and tested. In the temples, training to develop intuitive power was essentially scientific in its approach. The physical body was the laboratory. The student would examine each limb, each part, separately so that he could gradually build up a knowledge and awareness of the whole. The only way to know the body completely is to sense it. The temple exercises involved awakening the whole body. A certain spot would be pressed and the student would be required to explain precisely the reactions through his whole being; how the pressure had affected each organ and nerve. If the knee was touched how did it affect the solar plexus? the eyes? the roof of the mouth?

All healers should have an awakened intuition, available to bring through wisdom and knowledge. A fully awakened intuition suggests the awakening of the entire circuit, the linking with a network of energies which can contact and transmit signals at the speed of light. This is what we mean when we talk about a flash of intuition. At the speed of light we receive the appropriate information. We will know that our intuition is working when we are able to express accurate information about a stranger. In a flash something may come through. Or we may develop extra-sensory powers of smell, sight and hearing. We must realize that if information is coming through this is beyond the levels of smelling, seeing or hearing. We will not require clairaudience or clairvoyance. We must realize, too, that any knowledge coming through belongs to everyone. It is not our knowledge, it belongs to the collective consciousness. Intuitive knowledge comes through us, not from us; all we are doing is to bring it through. It should be said here that, ultimately, we, as healers, should be working for the patient, himself, to do the talking; in other words, for the patient to bring through his own knowledge and information. If the healer feels there is something particularly difficult and traumatic deeply rooted in a patient's past life he must sense what is the best thing to do. He must never bring through difficult or frightening things until the patient is ready for it, or perhaps he should recommend the patient consult somebody who has been professionally trained to deal with such things. We must never be ashamed to ask for help.

We can very easily waste our intuitive potential. If we employ our energies for making money; if we are ambitious and try to become well-known, we will have very little left for developing the highest levels. We have to build a pillar of strength inside us. Intuition becomes our strength and (in some measure) our security. We will know how to do the right thing at the right time. Through this pillar we can go up to any dimension. If we are unable to go in and build our own pillar we will forever have to dance round someone else's. As in the ancient dances we will be revolving round the totem pole of someone else's teaching: someone else will be our central focus. Long ago it was correct to turn outwards and look to a master for our development. But it was necessary for evolution that we should establish our individuality and, as we have seen, our mission in this era was to develop the main aspect of the individual, the intellectual mental aspect. This we have done too well. We have created the absurd world in which we live. In most people these days the intellect is so strong it imposes its will rather than serves the cause. We need now to expand its complementary opposite: the intuition. Energies and circumstances have changed and it is our mission now to find the inner teacher and bring through the intuitive knowledge that is within.

In order to awaken our intuition a channel has to be opened. It is important to realize that, just as our energies fluctuate, so do our intuitive powers, daily, weekly, monthly, yearly and in seven-year cycles and this applies equally to our patients. So we must be aware both of our own and our patient's lowest ebb.

In any serious attempt to develop the intuitive powers the ability to relax is vital. The first requirement is to be able to empty the mind of pressures and worries. Many healers will have had experience in past lives and will have worked to develop their intuitive faculties so that, even under difficult circumstances, even when they are tense – which makes the bringing-through of information difficult for most people – they are still able to open themselves and link up, thus enabling the intuition to flow. Most, however, will require a practical system of relaxation together, possibly, with techniques of boosting and amplification, which are dealt with later.

The second necessity for intuition is a change of brainwave, so that the circuit can gather the necessary power for raising the mind to higher dimensions and so that the information can be lifted from the collective consciousness or, as Jung calls it, the collective unconscious. This change of brainwave is the key to the intuitive levels, just as it is the key to healing, and we will be dealing with this later. Exercises for developing intuition will also be given later.

The indigo ray depresses the thyroid and stimulates the parathyroid, acts as a sedative, helps swellings, nose-bleeds, pain, haemorrhages, internal bleeding and insomnia.

Violet or Purple Ray

This is the ray of creativity. On this ray it is possible to heal using works of art. Art links mankind to the spiritual levels. It reflects his longing to go beyond his earth-bound realms. It is the expression of his innermost aspirations. Whatever its form it should enable a step from everyday consciousness towards another dimension.

In the temples, art was meant to spellbind those who

beheld it; it was meant to precipitate the beholder into a state of ecstasy beyond all boundaries and limitations. In ancient Egypt a creative artist would make something for an individual; it would be especially created and made potent for their use. In these days with mass production, objects have little or no healing potential, they can only reflect the radiations of their handlers and owners. If the latter are sick in any way the object will have sick radiations. The ancients knew how to infuse something with their energy-flow so that the work would always retain its healing vibration. We can still find this in many works of art, in sculptures, paintings and antiques which continue to radiate beautifully no matter who owns or touches them.

It is possible also to heal on this purple ray by using music, colour, crystals, movement, singing and fragrance. There is an important difference, however, between using these as tools and using them creatively. When we use these things creatively we help the patient, who may find it difficult when sitting in a room alone to find the necessary boost of energy with which to link to his higher self. We teach him how he can help to raise himself. The role of the healer on this ray, then, whether he uses colour or music or movement, is to encourage the patient to dance, to listen to music, to look at the colours in his house, even to paint: to inspire him so that he may aspire towards the highest levels. He begins to listen to beautiful music, to use colours creatively, to take up dancing and movement for himself. So this type of healer has reached the point at which he tries to stir the creative in people. He tries to bring out the creativity and inspiration in others.

This ray is good for headaches and, for some people, can be a slimming aid. It brings out the creative forces in us.

It might be helpful when we are trying to get an idea of these various levels to draw up a questionnaire. We might take a person and ask the following questions about him: is he sensual? Does he like games, sport, martial arts, digging the garden, washing floors? Is he active? Does he deal with ideas? Is he intellectual? Does he love animals, plants, the country? Is he protective and calming? Is he artistic? Does he paint, write poetry, compose music? There are so many ways of healing and we have to sense the various levels. This is the only way we can know them.

We have seen that energies may feel hot, cold or neutral. When people experience warmth, while being given healing, this means they are receiving red, orange or yellow beams and when they feel cool they are receiving the faster more spiritual rays – the greens, blues and indigos. Some healers emanate these spiritual radiations naturally. Some are more mental, which can be dangerous if you deal with hypnotic levels. A purely mental force can be misdirected. Some healers treat the human being as a kind of plumbing system. They imagine him as a dirty bath perhaps, something that needs to be cleaned in an ordinary everyday way, a chimney that has to be swept. Really it is better to give the person energy so that he can sort himself out. There is another point. If you act on a person's consciousness in order to influence it, it is an indication that you are not yet capable of making the link between your higher selves. In the highest realms of healing there is no element of drama or showmanship. The healer does not even need to use his imagination. He does not need to sit there imagining the patient all clean and healthy; in the highest realms all this will be taken for granted. On these highest levels the healer will be taking the patient home. Here is the essential difference between the levels of physical and spiritual healing. With spiritual healing you raise the consciousness of your patient in order to create possibilities. You do not take him over.

To be able to heal all the different types of illness is usually a case of progress, growth and evolution. If you are not a spiritual person there may be rays you are unable to produce and perhaps your patient requires these. Really we can only heal through our higher selves. The ego and the will do nothing. In America much research has been carried out as to the nature of healing energies. It has been observed that, in some cases, the personality does get in the way and that if the healer cannot get himself out of the picture, so to speak, and allow the force to flow through him there can be trouble. Thelma Moss cites a case of a healer who was working in the laboratory, voluntarily, and although he was

75

contributing greatly with his time and effort he was also enjoying the publicity that came with the work as well as the number of patients he obtained on a paying basis outside the laboratory.* One day a television company came to film the project. As usual the patient's radiation was photographed before and after treatment, using methods similar to Kirlian's. Before treatment the pictures revealed a deep-blue emanation, but after the treatment his emanations had all but vanished. In contrast the healer's pictures had increased in intensity after the treatment. Dr Moss suggests that the transfer of energy can travel not only from healer to patient but vice versa and may actually drain the patient.

Really it's only the higher forms of healing that will last and that can change the patient's attitude to himself. No man has the ability to create a cell from nothing, neither can he understand completely how it works. He can only add to, or subtract from, what has been provided by nature. By tuning into the highest levels all cells that have fallen out of their correct rhythm can re-programme themselves harmoniously. All over-activity will be removed, the patient will enter the spiritual dimensions, peace and well-being will sweep over him and the cells can mend their ways.

The Church has always maintained that it is God who heals, and that those who heal within the ministry act only as a channel for God. From the start it has always discouraged the realization of psychic gifts among its flock, one of the reasons being that these might be misused and exploited. Yet healing, as we have seen, is a natural exchange of energies. It would be perfectly acceptable for most people if we went along when they were ill and washed their floor, gave them a cup of tea and talked to them while they emptied their heart and got their grievances off their chest. If we jumped into a lake and saved them from drowning we would probably be given a medal, yet if we give them spiritual healing and save their life that way some people are nervous.

Providing a healer is professional, provided he is pure in

---

*See 'Photographic Evidence of Healing, Energy on Plants and People' by Thelma Moss, *The Dimensions of Healing*, Academy of Parapsychology and Medicine, Los Altos, California, 1972.

his motives, providing he tunes into the highest levels and becomes a channel, then it is his right to practise his gift.

Guides

At some point when we begin to give healing, or even before, we might contact a guide, or guides. Some of us may not be ready to take full responsibility for the healing and a guide may be necessary to advise and teach us. The early Christians who, as we know, were familiar with much traditional knowledge, often used guides. The idea was, as in divination, to contact intermediary spirits rather than communicating directly with God. St Paul, in his first letter to the Thessalonians, chapter 5, warns them 'to prove all things'. If a guide or a spirit appears we should always test it and if necessary reject it, but we should never ignore it. Guides can change according to vibrations and what is happening in our lives and we must be aware that just because someone no longer has a physical body it does not mean that he has automatically become enlightened. So we must always question any apparition or guide and ask, in the name of Christ, what it is. The highest guides will never seduce you in any way. They have gone beyond sex: there will be no sexual energy whatever involved in the contact.

Certainly guides can be a useful tool for raising vibrations but to a point we must bear in mind that we, as healers, must grow and develop and sometimes a guide will want to do the healing himself and take over completely. There is a difference between a guide who takes you over and does everything for you and one who stands back, only coming forward if you do anything wrong. It may not even be necessary to have a guide in the first place. Guides work through the same circuit as the healer and if the healer himself can raise his vibrations he does not need the support of a guide. It is best wherever possible for the healer to tune into his own higher self. It can be reassuring to have one or two guides around but they should be training us to stand on our own feet, teaching us to heal on our own. It is a common mistake to think that the guide is hovering about somewhere outside and so sit back, relying on him, when with enough determination and imagination we could get on with the healing by ourselves. Sometimes a healer imagines that someone is helping when really he is drawing on experience from past lives. The idea that he has a guide gives him confidence to get on with the job. Often guides are unable to get through in the first place. A healer may produce incompatible vibrations or have the wrong colours or he may not believe in guides anyway. In that case they will be unable to help even if desperately needed.

So if a healer does have a guide he should test him carefully and be aware that he should be learning to develop his own intuition rather than just following instructions. There is a real danger of being addicted to the guide and making no progress. Really while giving healing it is best to tune into love and cosmic energy rather than a guide no matter from which realm he comes. In any case the highest guides will make contact only with our higher selves, which is why it is so important to tune into this aspect. There are always times when we must be guided by our higher selves and we must never forget that our higher self is our friend who actually may have more colleagues 'upstairs' than we have down here on earth.

Pendulums

Once we can change our brainwave and tune into the intuitive levels we will be able to bring through information. Only a clear intuition can make the breakthrough to the highest levels but there are tools, as, for example, Professor Calligaris's system of plaque stimulation which can help bridge the gap and enable us to lift up, into the consciousness, information contained in the subconscious. Another tool is the pendulum which links the logical left brain to the intuitive right. We use the left brain, the intellect, to frame a list of relevant inquiries so that, with the aid of the pendulum, we may construct a comprehensive analysis. The pendulum can give a straight yes and a straight no; it can remain neutral or it can give a half-hearted yes or no. There are endless connotations and there is no limit to the information providing we pose the right questions. We can find out anything, from which foods are good or bad for us, which colours are needed, which vertebrae are out of alignment, to the location of mineral deposits in the earth, leylines, lost people and animals. But we must remember that the pendulum is only a tool for bridging the gap between the visible and the invisible. For the system to work we have to be competent dowsers in the first place and, like everything else, there is a danger of becoming addicted, of getting so used to relying on the pendulum that it becomes a habit. It is better to develop our own powers of intuition so that we do not have to rely on tangible props.

Psychometry

This is another technique for linking the visible to the invisible. In this case we generally obtain information by holding a physical object in the hand. So how does this work? We know that everything that occurs in the universe leaves a trace which cannot be erased, every event that has taken place remains imprinted on the ether. This film of life which records every action, every personal history, is continuous and available to anyone providing they have the key to enable them to lift the information into the consciousness. One of the gifts of a good psychic is to be able to slow down the film of life and look into the past. Holding an object in the hand and linking with it can be one of the ways of unlocking information. Whether we are researching into the history of an object, a human being or an animal, the procedure is the same. You change the brainwave, open the chakras and raise the energy levels, thus establishing a bond between yourself and the object you are holding. Be aware that you will probably pick up those facts about the object that interest you most. A historian, for example, will get a different point of view to a farmer. Let us suppose that we hold a stone and we are interested in nature: we might be taken back in time to the era in which the stone was created. If, instead, we are interested in history we might hold a stone

79

and be projected into a time in which either we ourselves have lived or in which we have a special interest.

Those who want to work with psychometry should be professional. When you hold an object in your hands you should be specific. What do you intend to examine? 'I am interested in the age of this object', you might say, or 'I am interested particularly in 55 BC'. You might then ask how many people during that year had touched the object. If you are unlucky there may have been hundreds, so again you must specify in which sort of person you are interested. Perhaps you hold a bit of harness worn by horses. You will probably pick up the horse, then you may pick up the people who used it and the places where the horse lived and worked. Eventually, through the various people who have touched it, an object can lead you to the history of a particular age.

Psychometry is something in which we should specialize. There is often a tendency for people to misuse it by trying to be a master of all trades. So if your interest is archaeology, stick to archaeology; if you want to study jewels, study jewels. Be aware that you will see things according to your level of energy. One person may hold a brooch and see it adorning a beautiful Greek woman, another does the same and sees it buried in a grave. The second person's psyche has gone immediately to a grave, the first to life and beauty, because this was their level of energy at the time. So if you feel low and you hold an object you may see a funeral rite while, if you feel cheerful and optimistic and you hold an object, you may get a marriage. It all depends on your energy at the time.

Psychometry is occasionally used for tracing lost objects. Again there is something particular to be aware of. Sometimes when we lose an article it was meant to go. It may be important for that energy not to be with us any more. So when things are taken away or stolen it can mean that we should not have the vibration of that article with us any more. We should think about this carefully before we go ransacking our psyches and the countryside.

4

The Healing Process

Much scientific research has been going on in Japan, England, Soviet Russia and the United States to find out what really does go on during healing. In the United States, especially, much effort has been put into mounting symposiums (under the auspices of such bodies as the Academy of Parapsychology and Medicine) with a view to informing the medical profession as to the scientific nature of modern psychical research or, as it is sometimes called, 'medical pioneering'. Healers have been studied in the laboratory by open-minded scientists and experiments have been carried out using plants, animals and enzymes as well as humans. Results have shown conclusively that healers do have the power to influence sick organisms and promote the growth of living matter.* In Soviet Russia where, until recently, healing was dismissed as unscientific, it is now widely discussed in terms of 'healing by biofield' or 'biofield influence', according to Larissa Vilenskaya, a Russian psychic researcher living in America who has published reports by the Washington Research Center, San Francisco.

So what does happen when healing takes place? We know first of all that no healer really cures anything. All he does is to give his patient a charge of energy so that the patient can heal himself. We know that this charge of energy brings the whole circulation to life so that the body can adjust and mend itself and, instead of weakening his immune system, the patient can begin to reverse the procedure and strengthen

*See 'Laboratory Evidence of the "Laying-on-of-Hands" ' by Bernard Grad and 'The Influence on Enzyme Growth by the "Laying-on-of-Hands" ' by Sister M. Justa Smith, *The Dimensions of Healing*, Academy of Parapsychology and Medicine, Los Altos, California, 1972.

it instead. Before we go into the mechanics there is a point to be made. With orthodox medicine the doctor may prescribe pills or liquid medicine as a corrective which in essence is nothing but encapsulated or liquefied vibrations. The help which we give by the laying on of hands is more rarefied. But perhaps the main difference between these two moderators lies in the assimilation. In allopathic medicine doses are standard and no attention is paid to individual requirements. Regardless of whether or not his system wants it, the patient assimilates the lot, sometimes with detrimental results. In the case of the subtle vibrations administered by the laying on of hands the patient will only absorb as much as he needs. Often during the session the force suddenly seems to switch off, indicating that the patient has received as much as is necessary.

Attunement

For healing to work at all a relationship has to be established rhythmically between healer and patient. We have seen that every individual possesses a biological clock which is tuned to the rhythm of universal movement; that human physiology is entirely dependent on rhythmic attunement with all things. When a person falls ill we know that he has fallen out of harmony with his basic rhythm. With a gesture of his hand, or even by his presence, the healer excites the molecular particles of the patient's body and provides an oscillation which restores harmony and brings order to chaos.

An essential to successful healing is to be able to change the brainwave to a receptive level of consciousness, to a state which could be described as 'dreamy'. This is an area which has exercised much research and machines have been developed to measure the brain reactions – Maxwell Cade has been outstanding in this field with his work in biofeedback. Numerous healers have been tested and it has been discovered that, when working with a patient, they produce a specific brainwave pattern which they impress on the patient, a pattern which the patient is unable to produce on his own without special training.

82

José Silva is among those who has researched into levels of mind and with the help of modern technology has created a technique for changing the brainwaves. His findings are interesting since they clarify the mechanics of attunement. His idea which he presents in the form of his mind-control course is that, when the brain resonates in the spiritual dimension, or at levels he refers to as Alpha, it is at its most receptive and can be used, among other things, for learning, contemplation, ESP and healing. It was discovered that at these levels the brain resonates at ten cycles per second, as opposed to the ordinary everyday dimension called Beta when it resounds at twenty cycles per second. To enable the mind to enter the spiritual dimensions easily he has devised the Alpha sound, a pulsatory rate, which he claims corresponds to the rhythm the brain produces when at these levels. By playing a tape of this pulsatory rate the brain will automatically fall in and resound to the rhythm. Equally, when the tape is played to two or more people, or to a whole group, the group's brainwaves should synchronize automatically, thus everyone will be in rapport, on the same wavelength. Silva is fond of remarking that at Alpha we pray for one another, at Beta we prey on one another. Silva claims also that the Alpha sound, when played on a tape-recorder, creates a magnetic field and if the tape-recorder is held over a diseased area of the body the resonance will penetrate every cell until they oscillate in harmony.

So the spiritual healer must be able to change his own brainwave and he must also be able to change the brainwaves of his patient so that both are on the same wave-length, pulsing at the same vibratory rate. For a short space of time their two systems will become as one, resonating, resounding harmoniously and the effect will have far-reaching consequences; each cell receives the ability to programme itself correctly once more. We know that real attunement is only possible if the healer can relinquish his personality, his ego, and all ideas of wanting the healing to be successful. Let us imagine a healing session. The patient enters all hot and bothered and the healer sits down beside him, his aura emitting a cool blue radiance. Gradually the patient cools down, absorbs the blue and changes, not because the healer is willing him to do so but because his emanations have calmed him down and both healer and patient have become one, they have become one with the high blue ray.

When two people are linked in this way it is as if they are connected by ley-lines. When two energies interact there will always be a birth of some kind, a creation, an inspiration. Forces start to pass between them and as the energies exchange and shine ever brighter other powers are drawn to them and eventually a great sheet of radiance appears. It is as if the whole of the cosmos shares in what they do.

So let us suppose that our healer meets someone who has a problem with his kidney. The healer tunes in and their auras come together. The patient's energy is able to expand away beyond himself, his mind will grow still, his brainwaves change and the vibrations rise. The full circulation begins to come to life and to release negativity, disposing of poisons. All the centres and organs oscillate in unison, pulsating, breathing, expanding and contracting harmoniously and gradually the kidney is restored to its regular rate. The patient is fortified and able to face up to life, able perhaps to let go of people, possessions, jobs and habits that are no longer necessary to him: able to change. Let us suppose now that a second patient has cancer of the liver which means that the cells of the liver are multiplying in a disorderly way and their proper programming is not functioning. The whole circuit will be affected by this one unharmonious organ. The patient will need cool blue and green energies which will act as a sedative and the over-activity of the liver cells will be curtailed.

We know that our bodies are a linked system of conduits and energy points and that the healing energies flow through these channels creating electrical charges capable of producing positive and negative properties. When a patient is receptive to the positive charges healing will be felt as warmth, the dormant areas of the circuit will be quickened and the blockages will be dissolved. The faster, cooler negative energies will engender a feeling of calmness and the overcharged areas will be smoothed out.

There is only one force and, as Edgar Cayce pointed out, its manifestations in man are electrical. A spark of electricity is God in motion. Know then, Cayce said, that force in nature that is called electrical, electricity, is that same force you worship as creative, or God in action.*

It is interesting here to cite the research that has been carried out into the electrical nature of healing energies by Canon Andrew Glazewski, theologian and physicist. He has found experimentally that a voltage applied to a certain place in any organism will affect the flow of fluid in the surrounding tissues and produce stress in the local environment. The patterns of such stress will differ from place to place in accordance with the structure of the tissue. The same voltage will produce a different stress pattern in the liver than in the adrenal gland and the supply of nutriments will be affected correspondingly. In disease therefore the abnormal electrical state of the affected organs will interfere with the circulation through them. A malfunctioning organ has a surplus of positive charges; if there is overcharging in any organ the blood stream will try to regulate it but if this does not work there is a surplus of positive ions, an overcharging which will affect the whole of the bloodstream.

The electrical state can be restored to normality by application of the healer's hands. The hand has its own electrical field which is especially strong around the tips of the fingers and when healing is given the palm will radiate strongly. Thus by approaching his hand towards the patient's body the healer introduces his own energy-field into that of the patient. Glazewski noted during his researches that any disturbance can be registered in the hands and that a severe disturbance can be felt further away than a minor one. The hand, he concluded, acts rather like a sponge and when introduced into the energy-field surrounding the patient will absorb the excessive charges.

So our hands are really antennae which are able to supply us with extra energy when we need it. They are able also to collect beneficial negative ions – which is why it is helpful to put them anywhere there is pain. They can disperse any accumulation of positive ions. Stretching the hands above the head is one of the best exercises we can do. This allows

*See *Edgar Cayce Readings* compiled by the Edgar Cayce Foundation.

energy to move up the spine and maintains a balance between the left and right side of the body. There is often a tendency in people who are angry to clench their hands. But as our systems start to become sensitive we will find we cannot afford to clench or tense anything. We must maintain a relaxed body. The person who holds on, who is tight-fisted with his energy on whatever level, whether it is money, information or anything else, will have problems which will be likely to manifest in his liver and spleen.

Making a Channel for Healing Energies

To perform any sort of psychic work we know that we have to tap into some source of energy. Sometimes it is necessary to amplify or to boost the system in order to open the chakras so that the higher voltages from the cosmos may be drawn down and channelled. We know that the ancients understood this and employed the radiation from stones, trees and sacrifices in order to boost their own. We know that shamans excite their energies by drumming and dancing. Another way to gather energy is through regular habit. If you sit down and study from 11am–1pm every day, for example, the required energy will start to flow automatically between these hours. Again when we begin something new this produces the necessary zest or drive with which to tackle it.

We have seen that it is possible for a healer to use earth energies together with his own electro-magnetic force but that the highest healings come through drawing down and processing cosmic energy. Healing cannot last or be entirely safe if we use the physical levels of energy produced by our own nervous system. It is not uncommon to come across healers who say that they feel drained and exhausted after giving healing. This is because they are not opening their centres and creating a channel for the energies to flow but instead are using their own physical energies. The physical and etheric bodies are the healer's tools and the first essential is that he should know how to open his chakras so that he can bring down the light, channel it into the appropriate rays and distribute it. To put it another way the healer must

86

be able to open up the top of his head like a chalice so that he can drink from the cosmos.

The simplest way of describing healing is to say that it is an exchange of energies. Ideally we should be able to exchange energy with everything and everybody. When we are able to exchange with everything we will be able to feel part of all things, all stones, plants, jewels and animals; no longer will we feel enclosed and isolated within our skins, we will be able to join with the earth, the wind, fire and water and be one with the elements. This is difficult in these days, we have so much pollution on the planet, so many sick plants, animals and people. So much of the environment is degraded. We have to contend with so many negative thoughts, both of our own and belonging to other people, that it is difficult to exchange and share in the real sense. If we were able to give and receive energies automatically we would feel 100 per cent better. Instead we have to keep closing ourselves down and blocking our vitality and our hearts, which thrive on sharing. Yet until our hearts can open well, until we see that for every person we hurt our own hearts will suffer, we will never be able to develop the full force of our healing powers. It is when the heart is fully open that it has enormous power to heal. All our wrong thoughts, everything that goes against the higher self will affect the heart.

So if we do not have centres that open easily we should meditate and work with relaxation exercises. We must relax the physical body and release the tension especially from the shoulders and the heart. Yawning and sighing is good for this. If your physical body is in good shape there should be few or no problems but if you do have pain or tension you have to look at your emotions; the root may lie here. Perhaps your emotions are holding a chakra closed. If it is not emotion then perhaps it is the mind. The chakra wants to let go and is fighting to get bigger, but you are holding on and your left brain is causing it to contract. In such cases what you are doing is to fight your own energy, your own chakra.

So it is important to know what the chakras are doing. Are they open or not? In some people they may open so naturally that their owners will not be aware of what is happening. In others they may only open under deep relaxation. Usually the sensation of a chakra speeding up or getting bigger is a feeling of expansion or heat, just as in a sexual climax one chakra will shift another to a point where the movement goes over a certain velocity. At this stage there is a change of brainwave and the person in question may feel light and slightly giddy.

Many healers start to give healing before they are ready and this can be dangerous and harm the centres. Once the chakras are open the feeling is beautiful. But you have to watch for problems. If you give healing and you have palpitations, either something is not opening or you have had too much to eat. Whatever it is there is something you should look at. If you feel intense heat anywhere, especially up the spine, this is a bad sign and you need more control. So it is good to watch the symptoms and know what they imply.

As the chakras start to open and energies move you may have indications. Because, for example, the body is used to erotic sensations when the base areas are aroused you may imagine you are feeling sexy, or you may have a sense of gathering, of stirring, in the solar plexus. Energy can collect here and manifest, not so much as a feeling of heat but as if light is flowing, a sensation which is neither hot nor cold. The abdomen and solar plexus gather power for the left-brain hemisphere as well as for the whole body and you may feel you want to eat more: indeed, your system may produce gastric juices. So you have to sense whether you really are hungry or whether it is your centres which are accelerating. So sense what is going on. Be aware too that as soon as you increase this chakra your ego will be stimulated, together with its instinct for survival, and you may feel exercised by insecurity and start trying to establish your assets financially, emotionally and so on. Be aware too that if you eat too much or think too much about food this can also quicken the abdomen which in turn will excite the lower chakras and you may think you need sex. These are all different ways in which our energies can affect us.

Most people will find that when the heart, which is the most important but, ironically, the most difficult centre, does open there is a very definite experience of love and warmth.

88

When the throat opens you will be able to pinpoint problems and people will be drawn to consult you and to ask for your advice. So it is good to look hard at your vehicle and discover what sort of feelings you have in its various parts. They will reveal to you whether you are able to help others, or whether you still have work to do on yourself.

When we are ready to give healing we should have no sense of overcharging but should feel quite relaxed, not only during the healing sessions but with life itself. We will start to get signs: the right person, the right book, the right word, the right idea, will come to us. So we must watch for coincidences. As we grow more sensitive we may become aware of electricity and experience sparks and crackling in our clothes or from the air. We may receive small electric shocks when we touch things: little explosions. Our hands begin to come to life and sometimes seem much larger, sometimes puffy. They too may become more sensitive and different colours will produce in them different sensations. It is good to experiment with coloured ribbons and notice the variations.

So to be able to create a channel for the healing energies a healer must know how to open his centres. He must be able to change his brainwave and create a link between the patient's higher self and the higher levels of love and wisdom.

It is often possible to tell if the energies are circulating well from the look of the healer. If he is giving a lot of healing he should appear much younger than his age and be stronger in body and spirit than the average person. If he appears old and tired it is likely that he is not closing down and cleansing properly.

If there is any trouble, any blockage in the body, it will mean that that particular area cannot transmit light. The physical body will soon let you know if you are not functioning properly, if you are giving healing when you are too tired or run down. It is possible to heal people, yet be ill oneself. Often healers who are ill can make others better. But we have to be careful. We have a duty to ourselves as well as to others. The chakras may be opening in order to help people, but *how* are they opening? If we are not using the energies well, we may slowly be damaging ourselves.

Bringing energy down through the top of the head does help the channels to clear; often healers feel clean and full of vitality after giving healing. But the first thing we should do is to work on ourselves, eliminate our poisons and purify our systems. In order to understand healing we have to understand ourselves. All initiations were exercises to develop the vital self-knowledge. It is of course difficult to know ourselves well but at least we should try to know what we are doing. Most of us have an unfortunate tendency to ignore our own weaknesses, never seeing ourselves as others do. We have to try to reach the point when we can see ourselves. Our own ugliness can be devastating. We have to find the compassion and love to accept the ugliness, to go through it and transform it to beauty. Just as it is difficult to know and to heal ourselves it is often difficult to help those nearest to us; we pick up emotionally all that they are suffering and perhaps we are not strong enough to transmute and lift them, to give them the necessary lightness so that they can rise above whatever is affecting them.

Self-Healing

The natural healing force should be used to heal and make ourselves as strong as possible. Self-healing is not only meditating and changing the brainwave so that our immune system can be strengthened but it is giving the body practical support and encouragement. Breathing exercises, movement, relaxation and introducing positive ideas into the consciousness must all play their part. As we grow older we may not absorb our food as well as we used to; either by using our intuition, or by dowsing, or by both, we must make sure our bodies have all they need, particularly the vital trace elements. If we do not have the correct balance of zinc in our bodies, just to take one example, this will cause problems that healing will not be able to restore.

A way to begin our self-healing is to make a list of all the things that are preventing us from being completely healthy. Once we have got that out of our system it is good to go for a brisk walk, in bare feet if possible, relaxing the feet, breathing

90

deeply, then returning home and taking a bath. After this we can rest on the bed. Now we should relax, change our brainwave and try to lose ourselves in the highest energies. It is a good idea to try to hand ourselves, our bodies and our minds, to the highest wisdom — we can call it what we like, the angels, God, the universal consciousness. Imagine ourselves standing in a great fountain, standing there being bathed in clean water, going beyond one's usual boundaries to our higher selves. The mind, after all, has no idea how to make the body healthy and it is only the higher self that can be of use. But handing over the body to the highest wisdom means accepting also the possibility that any illness may continue, accepting also the idea of death; this is really the only way that the ego with its survival instinct can be sublimated.

Good ideas repeatedly fed into the consciousness encourage us to become healthy. Our thought processes, instead of having a blocking effect through fear, will enable the dynamic energy to take its course. The mind is the builder. What we think may become crimes or may become miracles. As our mental powers dwell upon our invisible thoughts so they give strength to them and they become real. The story of Aladdin is interesting here. When Aladdin rubbed his lamp he produced a huge thoughtform, a huge genie, which would obey him. This was a clever way of mind control. The thoughtform was turned into a large servant who could fulfil all Aladdin's desires: everything he wished for became true. Most of us, when we are ill, are like Aladdin; we produce something and magnify it. But Aladdin's magnification was positive. It is the negative sort of magnification that makes us ill. We, human beings, can either create or destroy. We can either magnify something or shrink it. If someone has an inferiority complex and thinks he is inadequate at doing everything, everything he does is likely to be ineffective and in order to try and correct this, to make his presence felt, he may become over-assertive. Certainly someone who has negative ideas about his efficiency embedded in his subconscious needs to change his image. It would be a good idea for him to imagine himself bigger, taller, stronger altogether, able to deal competently with everything in life, able to cope with anything. Magnification is one of the tricks we can use in order to create possibilities. But we have to use it carefully or we may make something too big to handle, with which we may not be able to cope.

How Morals and Ethics Affect Our Abilities to Heal

Ideally, a healer should give up smoking and drinking, lead a good life and think carefully about himself, the instrument he is offering for healing. Often, as he develops, his dietary patterns will alter and he will turn naturally to a simple and plain diet. In any case he should try not to eat or drink too much, not to overdo sex and to keep his mind pure. All civilizations, whether ancient or modern, hold codes of behaviour from which we deviate at our peril. Not to stick to these codes ultimately pollutes the etheric and damages the physical. It is true of course that some healers enjoy a long life, do wonderful work and smoke and drink quite heavily. The cleansing effect of the healing may have kept them going and, in taking on other people's problems, they may not have bothered to deal with their own. Nevertheless, at some time or other they will have to bring their own problems to the surface and deal with them.

Sometimes difficulty with releasing negativity and poisons through the appropriate excretory zones is due to guilty secrets. All forms of suppression affect the excretory zones. The base areas coarsen in all those people who are inclined to anger or guilt, who steal other people's wives, husbands and possessions, and who are unable to talk about these things. So if an individual has an illicit love affair it is possible that his base centre might improve for a while, so might his area of assimilation – the abdomen. But the solar plexus will darken and become heavy. If a married healer falls in love with a person who vibrates rapidly there will be conflict. On the one hand he will long for the affair to be open while, on the other, there will be a desire to conceal it so that friends will be unaware of what is going on; thus his heart will be pulled in opposite directions.

Ultimately, we have to transmute our sexual urges into

pure love, transform the Greek *eros* to *agape*, the ego-love to cosmic love. Often our desire is basic, we long for a partner, we link into a kind of fairy tale dimension where we imagine a handsome prince or beautiful princess galloping into our lives to make everything happy ever after. The sexual energy is the vital fire that will fuel our breakthrough to the higher levels. At the base of the spine is the heart of the storm. There has to be a storm to release all the potential. We will never be able to break through to the higher levels if we are wishy-washy, if we do things in a half-hearted way. We have to have flare, verve, enthusiasm, courage, sparkle and dedication.

5

Development and Training

It is understandable that some doctors should be hostile to the idea of spiritual healing. After all, they have been obliged to apply themselves to a long and rigorous scientific training. They have invested many years and much effort and then people appear out of the blue, apparently with no training, and start curing without being able to give any reasonable explanation as to what they are doing. It is wrong to have the idea that healing is so spiritual that we do not have to learn anything about it. This approach will mean that we are ignorant of what we are doing and will be unable to explain it to anyone. This way there will be quite a number of people we will be unable to help since we ourselves will not know what is happening.

Life itself has often been a school for healers. Many will have endured great suffering. Many will have opened through unhappy relationships and personal loss and illness and will have reached a point at which they are ready to fulfil their mission on earth. During that time people will have come into their lives, teaching them, guiding them, helping them. But no matter how naturally any of us do anything it really takes years of training to bring out the best. If we think we can perform miracles without making any effort to improve ourselves, sooner or later we will be faced with a test, we will be confronted by someone who cannot be healed. All healers should be ambassadors of their art and capable of answering questions. No one can be a really good healer unless he is prepared to study and practise for many years and to back up his gift with medical and spiritual knowledge.

First and foremost the motive of a healer is important.

94

What is in his mind? What is his motive for wanting to heal people? We must realize that, when we give healing, we use forces which act at subconscious levels and we therefore create a deep bond with our patient which makes him vulnerable. As healers we must not look for results, nor must we interfere. We must work only through the highest levels and above all we must beware of pride and vanity. We may achieve a certain success, enjoy considerable influence over others who may admire us greatly but we must never let this go to our heads.

The way to develop is to learn deep relaxation and meditation; learn to understand the body, movement and what counselling means; learn how to bring information through from another person. The patient must ultimately be responsible for his own system, so he must be helped to help himself, to do things on his own so that he will not be dependent on his healer.

Cleansing

The first essential is for the healer to keep his own centres and his aura as clean and as pure as possible. We know that the act of healing is in itself purifying and that some of the energies the healer brings down will help him to dissolve any coarse etheric particles he may have accumulated. The body is always inclined to store waste matter and the ancient yogis and masters went to great lengths to eliminate poisons, using techniques that seem extraordinary to us. When emotions are out of control it means usually that the blood is polluted, so it is important to cleanse the bloodstream.

Blaming others is a sure sign that cleansing is necessary. If we ourselves or our patients keep blaming everyone and everything for the problems of life, it is a clear indication that we are physically low and we need to cleanse. As we start to purify dingy vibrations will flow out of our consciousness by way of our mouths. The throat is one of the main clearing areas of the body and inability to exhale well is one of the basic causes of illness. Most of us use only one fifth of our lungs. Sometimes playing an instrument can help, the flute, perhaps, or the recorder. So if your exhalation is poor, blow things out as much as you can, blow out invisible candles or whistle. It is as important to purify the lungs with deep breathing and to do exercises to release the tension in the body as it is to eat the right food and to drink water.

Water is marvellously cleansing. If used correctly its healing properties will help us all our lives. Still waters will calm us; rivers, streams and oceans have a purifying effect and the sound of moving water can be mesmeric. Washing the feet raises the energy levels by cleansing the etheric – the vibration from a healer's feet are vital to him because through them he not only channels energy but releases a lot of dirt. Digging in the garden is very cleansing, the earth will absorb any negativity.

One way of cleansing is to immerse ourselves completely in others. If we wash people's floors, do their shopping and see how much worse off they are than ourselves it may help us to get our own problems into perspective. Most people who are ill are trapped in themselves, trapped in their pain and their worries; if we can find other people's pain and worries more important than our own we may begin to attract people to us who can help us through our own ordeals.

The lungs and the colon are connected and if people are not able to release negativity it means that either they are not exhaling properly or they are not voiding through the excretory zones. Frequent emptying of the bowels helps dispose of the rubbish from the physical and etheric bodies. But in order to let go we have to relax. Energies change through evolution and the excretory area in these days is starting to shrink. In other words it is more difficult to let go nowadays. Our forefathers had large excretory chakras and negativity was able to pass through easily. Every time we excrete we should release all our unwanted thoughts and ideas, we should literally pull the chain on our minds and let everything go but, in this twentieth century, constipation is a common problem. Again, our forefathers crouched – as many 'ethnic' peoples still do – and so automatically relaxed this centre. But modern lavatories are not helpful and actu-

96

ally allow energies to collect in the lower part of the body. Constipation often starts at an early age with 'potty training'. This is sometimes carried out in such a way as to upset the child with the result that his bowel or bladder movements are inhibited. The result will be disharmony in the base chakra which resounds through all the centres and may affect him for the rest of his life.

Often we need to re-educate our patients in their approach to diet, exercise and breathing. The home environment of the patient is important. If we send a patient back having given him healing and there is a bad energy in the house or environment this will probably cause the problem to recur. When any of us walk into a bad environment it can affect various organs. We can make ourselves ill because a room has imposed upon us and our movement. So it may be necessary to work on the environment. Spring cleaning, using crystals, beautiful music, incense – there are many ways to purify a house. Warn your patients to look at the trees in the district and in their gardens and see if there are any strange growths; discover, too, if there are any negative streams. Negativity in the earth can cause problems.

Some people are natural losers of energy and this happens more readily when people are ill. Sometimes you find people on their death-beds giving all their energy to visitors. So if two people walk in and one looks radiant and the other seems exhausted, be careful how you judge them. The person who looks exhausted may have cleaned and charged up the other person. So if a patient keeps coming to you for healing you must consider whether it could be his family conditions which are causing the trouble. Unless his environment is cleared the patient will keep being exposed to the negativity that caused the problem originally and will be unable to progress.

If your patient leaves uplifted but then starts again smoking, drinking or eating too much, and over-indulging in sex, his illness will come back in another form. The healing is meant to change his mind and his way of life and to awaken his consciousness.

Some healers are vulnerable to their patients' conditions, so be careful that you do not take your patients' illnesses into your body rather than transmuting them. In clearing others this sometimes happens and if we do not clear our aura well we too may become ill. Remember we are responsible for our auric space and we have to make it beautiful. If people come to us and are healed immediately and at the same time we feel strong and buoyant and our body is healthy, probably all is going well. A healer who cleanses and purifies may find that he changes the whole pattern of his life. Above all he should be oriented to spiritual progress and to accomplish this perhaps he needs to meditate more and gradually cut out of his life everything that stops him from developing his true potential.

Relaxation

Relaxation of the physical body is vital: it is as important for the healer as the patient. Inability to relax is often one of the reasons that poisons accumulate in the body. Aside from this an essential for healing is that both healer and patient should be able to relax all tension and it may be necessary for us to work and perfect our own relaxation techniques before we teach them to our patients.

One of the best ways of relaxing physically and releasing energy is to make each toe and each finger move in circles. Turn them to the right and to the left. Then you can do the same with the wrist, the elbows, shoulders and feet, turning them all in both directions. Pull the fingers and toes gently, take the arms and giving them a little pull. Emphasize these stretching mechanisms in your mind, imagine your arms and legs getting longer and longer. You can say to yourself, 'I am stretching my fingers, my toes, my neck', so that if you do not care to stretch yourself physically you can use the mind instead. If you have a tense part hold that part with your hands and in your mind and emphasize the wholeness, the health, of that part. Tension can be like an armour and we can breathe into that armour seeing it gradually get softer and softer until it evaporates and disappears.

A relaxed vibration depends on the things around: lovely things and lovely colours are more relaxing than ugly ones.

A good way to approach relaxation is to imagine going into a warm, restful house or lying on a sunlit beach, walking through a spring meadow or a shady wood. Everyone has a different place in which they like to unwind. If you are very tense and are indoors it is as well to start with physical measures. A warm luxurious bath might be helpful. Give the body a good rub afterwards and it will bring it to life while at the same time feeling peaceful inside. So snuggle down and find a comfortable place. Nestle a little and then stretch the body. Make this something very definite. Have a good stretch. Stretch your legs out and stretch slightly on the diagonal, a really good stretch. Once you have stretched you will be able to relax much easier. If for any reason the stretching, the bath, the snuggling down in a restful place, does not work then try clenching. Start by grinding your teeth, then smiling, laughing, sighing, yawning, then try to feel the whole of your face relaxing, allow the shoulders to lift, bring them down, relax them, grip your hands very tightly. Then very slowly, finger by finger, just let go and then do the same with the legs, curling in the toes, stiffening the legs and very slowly letting go. Contract the buttocks and the abdomen really hard on a good exhalation and then very slowly let those parts go as well.

All these are ideas to relax you. But you have to get your mind to rest and lie down as well. You must avoid lying there thinking about what you are going to do next – the shopping or rearranging your life. If there is any tense part in the body or mind this means you have not completely relaxed.

So in the beginning meditation is really only relaxation. Remember that the physical body is the vehicle which can take us through to the highest levels. It has particular gates of consciousness which can open and lead us to the highest. As we know, the etheric body backs the physical and if we disobey the natural laws it becomes dark and heavy. Really our whole body is a map of consciousness. The first thing that happens when we sit quietly, relax and change our brainwave is an interaction with the cosmos, with the galaxies and planetary systems, which produces an influx of energy. The whole chakra system starts to quicken. Relaxation and quickening should come together. There are some people who react in the opposite way and slow down in meditation – this is because they have a lot of sorting out and clearing to do – but most speed up, their energies spin round faster and faster like the propellers of an aeroplane. Sometimes we can get prickling sensations in various parts of our body which means that small parts of energy have opened and have started to release light. It is possible for some healers to have such power that they have burnt a person. Madame Kulagina in the USSR on several occasions actually set her clothes alight.*

Meditation

The purpose of meditation is to enlargen the centres and to raise the consciousness. Like driving a car along a motorway we accelerate faster and faster, changing into top gear as we do so. Really our whole system is geared for lift-off. All we have to do is to train our minds and focus the energy properly. Even if we just sat and thought how beautiful life is; how marvellous it is to be able to sense and appreciate, it would be surprising to find the level of energy we could raise. Meditation is linking rather than thinking. Remember our minds are the builders: we become what we create. If we consciously make ourselves into a channel we will transmute more energy. If we introduce something large into the mind it will have the effect of magnification which produces more energy so that we can change gear and reach higher levels.

Every time we meditate we change the cellular structure, freeing it from body and emotions and connecting it to the higher levels. Meditation is really a journey home: we begin to sense our true reality and composition. Often our problem is that we are unable to go home enough. We cannot return to that still sanctuary deep inside us which is the only place in which we really can be secure.

We live in such a busy environment with so much to distract us that it is difficult to still our minds and to empty

*See *To the Light* by Lilla Bek and Philippa Pullar, Unwin Paperbacks, London, 1985.

100

them. Yet this we have to do; it is essential for removing all those mental blocks which restrict circulation. Learning to concentrate and control the mind will improve our ability to live more fully in the present, neither regretting the past nor worrying about the future. Thus our vital energy will not only be conserved but directed economically. Try as an exercise to look at an apple or a flower for a certain span of time, controlling the mind so that your thoughts do not wander.

Meditation will act upon us according to our thought patterns so we must recognize and release all negative ideas. It cannot be reiterated too often: we are what we think. The last thought before we go into meditation is most important since it creates the mood of the meditation. The quality of our breathing will also influence the meditation. Sometimes it is difficult to sit still and be quiet. This is where the tools of the trade come in: prayer, mantras, breathing exercises, visualization. In the temples they used all kinds of techniques for controlling the mind and body, developing awareness and raising the consciousness: music, mandalas, sacred movement among them. There were special exercises for projection. For example, a place would be selected, a temple or a garden, you would enter your meditation, breathe deeply and visualize the selected place. The exercise might be to detect an article which had been put physically into the selected spot and you would have to find it. In other words, you had to project yourself with your mind so strongly that your projection became real.

Some people find it helpful to construct, mentally, an inner sanctuary in which to work. José Silva suggests that his students build a laboratory complete with all the equipment they will need for their psychic work. We may need symbols that the psyche can understand so that the mind can rise to the highest intuitive levels. The boat in the water is always a symbol of transcending from one level to another and the island is an important symbol which allows us to reach our higher selves. All symbols of roads and paths heighten intuition and link us to our spiritual journey. The tree of life, water, mountains, plants, ladders, spirals, all these, as techniques, can help us raise our consciousness. There are times when spontaneously we can go very high, times when we release a huge volume of energy, but there are also times when the mind has to be stilled, the physical body dealt with, and then these techniques have to be used. We have to ask ourselves what is best. Eventually we have to progress even beyond symbols and, by opening the third eye, begin to look into what has hitherto been invisible. There is a whole world out there of which most of us are oblivious. In meditation we should be like a beam of light, a lens which is projected into time and space so that eventually we can deal with levels of which we have probably never even dreamed.

Without concentration and contemplation meditation can be rather empty. Monks used to end their day by making a list of their inadequacies, getting them out of their system that way. But self-exploration can be painful, it requires courage. So many people live their lives without knowing themselves. Embarking on self-exploration means daring to look in the mirror and seeing not just a doll but a real human being with all his faults. So many people have a plethora of faults about which they know nothing: they live their lives without knowing themselves: they are blind. Contemplation brings the dregs to the surface. Never be ashamed. Seeing yourself in a clear light with all your faults and failings can be very painful. Meditation can take you down to the very roots of your instability and this may take a long time to deal with. How on earth, you may wonder, can such a mess help others? We have to watch ourselves and our habits. The physical body will usually react first. If your shoulders are wrong, indeed if any part of you is wrong, it will surface. Remember that if we are going to experience higher voltages through the body we need it to be perfect. So, as you sit in meditation try and be aware of what your body is trying to tell you. If you start needing to swallow, or your tummy starts rumbling, your throat needs to clear, you start sneezing, this means that these areas are starting to open. Some of the best meditations are those in which the physical body starts to realign, shoulders go up, necks stretch. Really, meditation is sitting still and allowing the body in that quiet and stillness to work out its problems. Our forefathers did this at night; in these days people are so tense when they

102

sleep that the body cannot cope. It has not finished its work by the time that it wakes in the morning.

We have to be aware that, as we grow sensitive, we will begin to react to the environment more. People have even been known to grow allergic to their husbands and friends. An underground stream running beneath your house can make your meditation stronger but, if the waters are not pure, it may do the opposite. If you have an aura that accumulates easily and does not release, you may not become stronger at all, you may stiffen up and become arthritic. So be aware that meditation can make you more sensitive. We have to ask ourselves: are we stronger than our environment, or is the opposite true? Those of us who affect the environment least are the ones who have most work to do on themselves.

Meditation should be a friendly, warm and beautiful time. But if you have not put your heart into your meditation, nothing will happen. Everything you touch, every heart, every animal, everything in nature, all your belongings and possessions, should rise to a higher level. We must try to sense how much we are in control. We must become more sensitive to the seasons, planets, the earth itself, so that eventually we can become part of everything. We need to be creative and to be creative we need to be fired, we need the fire of the universe: the energy of the base chakra. So try to sit in meditation and tune into this fire and think again how beautiful life is.

Never push yourself. Take meditation gently. If nothing happens today, try again tomorrow. Just observe: try to balance yourself, see whether your heart slows down, whether your solar plexus feels overactive. Watch your symptoms. Do you feel any form of tension or sensation? You may need to yawn and exercise your face. As we sit in meditation all the pulses inside will change and become alive. If you have any area that is giving trouble you can concentrate on the spine and the link between the chakra and the organ and try to create a harmonious rhythm balanced by the breath which will help dissolve the problem. The chakra system can be helped by deep relaxation. As we know, some-

103

times one centre opens quicker than another but the balance within the centres must be maintained. Relax and think of each one of the chakras in turn: relaxing and letting go. Just as our digestive system should function spontaneously and easily, so the chakra system should be easy and spontaneous.

The adept will eventually be able to take full responsibility for everything he has done. He will not blame his father, mother, teacher, husband, wife, friends and neighbours for everything he has been doing wrong. He will realize his need for these people in his life to help his development. Gradually, interesting things start to happen. The right person appears, the right group to help and heal him, the right idea. Things will clarify. The direction of his path, his vocation in life will emerge.

The first step towards mind over matter is being able to control ourselves. We start with ourselves and the control of our lives so that we are not forced into situations and circumstances we can neither understand nor cope with.

The Healing Room

We have first of all to prepare the healing room. This should always be kept as clean as possible. It should be a place where peace prevails and from which everything negative is removed. When we have one person after another coming to be healed we must know how to empty and cleanse it – preferably after each patient. Burning a candle and/or incense helps to clean the room during and after healing. It is helpful, too, for the room to be painted blue, green, apricot or white, and to keep it full of things that radiate well: beautiful pictures, crystals, fresh flowers. We must remember that all patients need to feel relaxed and safe and so the room must feel comfortable to them. So we must be aware of the space around us and imagine how patients will feel upon entering it.

Preparation of the Healer

We need to give ourselves time to relax before starting our healing session in order to open our hearts as much as possible. Some work well after a meal which earths them so that they feel secure and happy about rising to high levels. Others will find a meal makes them too heavy. Whatever the case, healing always works better after a good stretch. So to ensure that you can be a really good channel always stretch and lengthen yourself in order for the energy to be able to flow through freely.

So the healer must try to relax his whole body and, in order to release any tension, check right the way through from top to toe, without forgetting the hands, arms, neck and shoulders. He should also use the cleansing breath (see Appendix II) to strengthen the auric space and to help the body release poisons. He may also focus his mind on words such as 'love', 'peace', 'joy' and 'well-being'. The more deeply he is able to relax, the higher his consciousness will be raised.

Preparation of the Patient

When people come to be healed they may know nothing of meditation. Perhaps the only things they can concentrate their minds upon are their own illness and unhappiness. So the healer has to help them to change their mind and to be comfortable. Ideally this should happen automatically. The healing room should be so full of strong vibrations that, just by coming into it and sitting there quietly, a patient feels quite different, without being able to explain why. The sounds emanating from the healer's aura should also be able to balance and renew those coming from the patient so, as soon as the patient walks in, harmony should begin to reverberate.

First of all, the healer should discuss with the patient what his problems are. Then, before the healing begins, the patient must be earthed. He should be told to think of his feet as being very heavy; the healer may suggest to him that his feet are like magnets holding him down. An interested patient will probably want to be involved in the healing act so, at an appropriate moment, the healer can teach the patient to relax and to sense his own body-consciousness, to sense where he is holding on to stress or tension and how to release

105

it through the feet and the out-breath. If the patient is very tense it may be necessary to spend some time meditating with him, perhaps using some form of creative visualization or playing some soothing music. We must remember that relaxation of the patient is absolutely vital. If the patient is unable to relax it is unlikely that healing will take place. In any case it is good to allow the patient to sit quietly and try to feel whether the radiations in his feet are getting stronger, whether warmth or coolness is flowing into his body. Every person is different and we should tune into their individual requirements which may vary every time they come. Try to get the patient to tune into his higher self. If he is religious he should be encouraged to link with God in some way or to say a prayer. If he is interested in meditation he should be helped to meditate at home.

The Healing Act

As the healer prepares to heal he may notice changes occurring within himself. He may stand more upright, he may breathe more easily and become calm and peaceful. If he feels he is changing inside, yet nothing around him has been affected, then he should be suspicious. The whole atmosphere should change.

Technique

The healer's technique will be a question of his individual judgement and development. It is up to each healer to develop an effective way and, at the same time, not to get trapped into habits. One way to approach the patient is to link with his highest aspect – that aspect that knows exactly how to make a cell healthier. In some cases the two higher selves will link up and the healing will take place wordlessly. Some patients, however, need words. They are uneasy with silence and it would take a very strong healer to create the right vibrations for them to feel comfortable. So sometimes it is appropriate to talk to the patient during healing; he can then respond and an exchange of energies will be established in this way. Certainly it is important to know whether or not the patient needs to talk. Some patients are not sensitive and have no way of knowing they are receiving healing.

The following is a guideline, a procedure, with which to work during the laying on of hands.

First, stand with your hands placed lightly on the shoulders and tune into your patient. Many healers like to start with the feet. The point is that there are special energy centres on the shoulders and, as you touch these, the feet will also release and relax. So placing the hands on the shoulders and tuning into the patient will help to relax the whole of his body. So spread your hands across the shoulders and tune in. We must never go barging into a person's energy-field without first asking his permission. So it is good manners first to ask permission silently from the patient's higher self before proceeding. This can be done either by keeping the hands on the shoulders or holding them for a moment above the patient's head. Next link into the aura and tune your own and your patient's energies to the highest levels. You can imagine white light or you can tune into the highest archetypes, Christ, Buddha, the angels, and say a silent prayer to them invoking their help. So never begin without tuning into these levels or you will only be giving the patient physical healing rather than spiritual, which means that parts of the patient's body may not be able to heal. Remember that, on the highest levels, you, yourself, do nothing except raise the patient's consciousness in order to create possibilities. The less you do the better. The less of you there is, the more there will be of the highest levels. So tune into the highest levels and let them flow down. Putting your hands on the shoulders also has the benefit of allowing much of the tension that may have gathered there to release. The neck and shoulders are areas which collect a great deal of pressure and it is wise before working on the heart to relax the back of the neck, the shoulders, down the arms to the hands. You should be able to feel the patient responding and a lovely sensation of peace descending.

Some people place their hands directly on the body, others use the aura during the laying on of hands. If you keep your hands a few inches from the body your energies will be absorbed into both the physical body and the auric space, in other words, they will be absorbed by all the bodies, but, if you keep your hands only on the physical body while you give healing, the energies will be absorbed on this level alone which means there are not so many possibilities. The important thing is that changes must occur on all levels. Actually, for spiritual healing it is not necessary to touch the body at all but some people will not believe that anything has happened unless they have felt some physical contact.

So, starting with the top of the head try scanning down the body with your hands held a few inches away from the person. This will calm the aura then, if necessary, you can return to any particular area and give contact healing. Do not immediately put your hands on the place where the pain is experienced but scan the main areas, forehead, throat, heart, solar plexus, abdomen and reproductive zones. If you are sensitive you may also be able to notice if the shoulders, ankles or hip centres are not functioning properly. Just as it is wise to work on the neck and shoulders before dealing with the heart so it is good when you cope with the lower areas to work also on the hips and feet. If the region needs only a little balancing then all you have to do is to keep your hands there for a few seconds.

You may have a patient who vibrates so fast that their physical body is unable to function, they may be open all the time and have problems. Again you may have a person who is the opposite, he is closed up, unable to release and his energy becomes stagnant and dark – often it is the nice people who, not wanting to hurt others, tend to shut things away inside themselves. You may have patients with some parts going too fast and some too slow. The whole point of healing is adjustment and balance. Sometimes you may pick up when a centre is losing energy, sometimes you may not, but never stop trying, never limit yourself by sitting back and saying: 'I'm not the sort of healer who can do this or that', never feel you're not making progress. If you are unable to do something this means you need to take yourself in hand and do more work on yourself. Meditate more. So try to use your intuition and feel where the healing is needed, rather than relying on the patient to tell you. Remember that

108

the area that appears to need treatment most is sometimes
not the source of the problem. Perhaps it was some trouble
in the kidneys that created havoc in the other organs and
eventually pain manifested in the bladder. It will not be
enough to put your hands only where the pain manifests.
You have to deal also with the kidneys.

So scan the body by running the hands one in front and
one at the back, monitoring the energy-fields. You should
feel if there is too much agitation, if the chakras are fast or
slow. In the beginning one can only hope for these two
extremes: feeling that a chakra is not sending out any energy
or feeling that it is over-charged. Scanning the body should
be like playing scales on a piano, each chakra ascending or
descending on a slightly different note. So go down the body
looking for signals. Every healer has different signs. Some
people may get tingling in the hands, some even get
sensations in the elbows. Lilla finds that the roof of her
mouth lifts. Sometimes you can tell when a chakra is too
open: you have a feeling that the patient is unearthed. Be
aware that if you keep suspecting that something is wrong
in a certain area – if all your patients seem to have something
wrong with their throats, for example – you could be
reflecting some problem you, yourself, hold. Be aware, too,
that what you see at any one time may be the pattern of
your own growth which is reflected back from the other
person.

After this most people work by instinct. Balancing out the
patient's body should be intuitive. Healers work in different
ways. Some see colours, some hear sounds, some receive
flashes of information. There are all kinds of different
approaches. When help comes through the higher self we
need to do very little apart from working down the body.
You will reach a point where you will be guided as to your
actions so that the patient's own release mechanism can
work. We have to put the patient in the light, but the light
will not be able to travel properly unless the blockages are
released. Sometimes if there is a stopping in the chakras it is
helpful to rub or massage that area gently, but it is not good
to employ circular stirring movements over any part of the
body either with the hand or the pendulum. Human beings

are not like machines, we should not tighten or unwind any of their parts, but give them the energy to do it themselves. If a healer's hands are healthy he will probably find he has no problems with his healing. In any case it is good to rub the hands to discover whether or not they are linked. You may feel a point at which they do not connect. When you are healing and one hand is in front of the patient's body and the other is behind, the stronger the attraction between the hands the more it will help the patient's flow of energy.

Earthing for both healer and patient is vital. Look at any electrical gadget and you will see it has a fuse and an earth to stop too high a voltage from passing through it and causing an explosion. In the same way and for the same reason we have inner fuses and an earthing mechanism which acts through the feet. Many people who are ill do not have good earthing equipment. Some are completely unearthed and have far too much energy over the top of the head. Such people are accident-prone, fearful, over-sensitive and often create illness through their imagination. Others go too far the other way: they are too heavy, too absorbed in their lives and in materialism, they over-indulge in all the good things of this earth with the result that they build up too much energy in their feet and are unable to release it.

It is so important in any healing that the unhappiness of the patient should discharge. Let us suppose that a patient comes to you who is really depressed and his unhappiness is affecting his liver. Just putting your hand on his liver is not going to be the answer. Until the heart can empty its sorrows and frustrations the liver will not get better. Crying is a marvellous liberation and should always be allowed to continue. Stretching and yawning are also good for getting rid of strain. We have to be aware, too, that certain diseases require more release than others. When dealing with cancer, for example, we would normally be drawn to the heart and the coccyx. We have to work to clear both these areas.

We will know when the healing is completed; usually the energy seems to switch off. The amount that is accepted depends on the patient's higher self and on how much his body can receive. When the healing is finished we must learn to detach ourselves from the patient or we will maintain a

110

bond, a cord, between the two of us and our own energy will be sapped. We have to learn to close both ourselves and our patients down. So, when the healer has finished, he should ask the patient to become aware of the feet. We may need a symbol, a password for the psyche. We can use flowers, perhaps, candles, or special clothes which we assume for healing and take off when it is finished. Repetition is the key. Repeat your closing ritual again and again until it is firmly engrained in your subconscious. Finally, it is a good idea to wash your hands, preferably in cold water. Two electric circuits have come together and you need to break the contact and regain your own circuit.

Working with Other Healers

If you feel that you lack in strength or confidence, if you feel you do not have the required courage, it is often helpful to work with others for the support and the extra charge of energy. When three or more are gathered together a small chakra or centre of light is formed. Be aware, though, that patients can accept only a certain amount of healing energy. Imagine someone who is getting on in years being stormed by powerful charges from several healers. Although his system will stop him from absorbing too much, so much force is not really going to be of much benefit. Sometimes it is necessary to have men and women working together, but they must be mutually well balanced so that their radiations fuse harmoniously. Two healers working together often miss out a little, each should be aiming to gather his own spiritual strength and not depend on another. Some patients find it disturbing to have two or more healers operating on them simultaneously and probably most of us would prefer to tell our troubles to one person rather than a crowd.

When people are drawn into a healing partnership generally there is one who is stronger and who helps the others to learn. Gradually such apprentices should be encouraged to give as much healing as possible by themselves so that they may develop.

111

Absent or Distant healing

To understand how absent healing works we have to consider again the universe and its interacting weave of cosmic energies. It may be helpful to imagine the texture of a piece of cloth, the warp and woof, some strands lying harsh and thick, some finer and softer. Now imagine this fibre stretching through the universe connecting all matter, whether visible or invisible, joining every nerve to every organ, linking every soul to every other soul, every soul to every planet and so on. When healing is sent to someone at a distance, thought is projected which travels down the fibres of our imaginary web, bringing people together. This is an example of the whole circuit, the microcosm and macrocosm, flashing into action. Every cell and every organism is part of this universal loom into whose mesh we engage when we send distant healing. This is the same network that was originally used by our forefathers for survival, for sensing the approach of danger. All we are doing is working on a larger scale and, instead of receiving energy, we are using the system to project healing radiations. In this way it is possible to send healing to a person on the other side of the world. Thoughts flash like lightning through the web and links are created. You think of something in Camberley and in the twinkling of an eye it affects someone in Calcutta. Our forefather's cognizance of the network of telluric currents is significant here. During the Romano-Gallic wars the Romans were astonished by the fact that the least of their movements were immediately apprehended by the enemy. This raises the suggestion that the Celts, who were celebrated for their traditional lore, used the ley-lines rather like our modern telephone cables: they were engaged in transmitting thoughts, in the telepathic transference of information.

Be aware that, if you are working alone sending healing telepathically, it helps for you to get the timing right, in other words it helps to know the best time to send healing. We all have times at which different organs switch on, times when our energies are stronger than at other times. So, when conducting healing, we have to try and arrange a time when the patient is at his most receptive. People who are inclined to be intellectually oriented find it difficult to pick up energy from healers during the day; at night in the darkness the right side of the brain brings more sensitivity, so it is easier to heal such people in the evening. Others may be tired at night and it will probably be better to send healing to them early in the morning, but all this will depend on yourself and how relaxed you are.

Once you have cleansed and purified yourself you can send healing while lying down; you will be able to go higher in your consciousness if you earth your body, imagining that your feet are firmly on the ground. Another way of sending healing is to leave a list of names in your sanctuary. Providing the place in which you lodge them has been put in the light these people will also be held in the light and certain energies will be given to them. These are different ways in which we can serve. Certain people do well when healing is sent to them telepathically, others need the reassurance of someone physically with them.

It is not necessary for the patient to believe or even to know anything about the healing, although it is best if he himself asks for help and, if he can tune in consciously knowing what hour the healing is going to be given, this too is beneficial. In any case the amount of healing he can absorb will only be that which his higher self desires, that which is right for him. With absent healing, just as with contact healing, we should take the patient closer to his higher self; he may receive ideas to visit an osteopath or to purify himself with herbs. Ideas to help him to be more creative may come to him, or he may simply feel reassured that someone cares and be fortified into believing that he can get better.

Working in a Group

Transmitting healing through exerting group energy is more powerful than working individually, but it requires a different technique. When a healer operates by himself he will cord himself to the patient to whom he is directing the healing. A group does not function like this. Indeed it would be quite wrong if a whole group were to cord to one person.

Usually a list of names is prepared of all those requiring healing. Since it is difficult to think of many people simultaneously, people's names are read out individually, each person on the list receiving the group's attention in his turn. The group will sit in a circle and as a name is called the person is imagined there in the centre of the circle being bathed in a fountain of light. The group will probably tune into the vibration that each name releases in the room and healing will be dispatched to that person. Sometimes a bowl full of names is placed in the middle of the circle and everyone concentrates on that without the names being uttered. The healing effect of these two techniques is slightly different. The whole group concentrating simultaneously on one person is in effect more intense than when the focus is on a bowl of names, in which case the energies will be more diffused.

Group meditation is important. It binds the group together and helps the members to lose their individual egos and blend into the collective consciousness. Group energy is powerful and helps to make the building, where the meditation is held, vibrant, also the surrounding land. The linking of so many auras produces a beam of light round the house whose bright radiations will be able to dissolve any negativity.

All these techniques are only suggestions. If you have been working with one method for a long time you will have conditioned your psyche to operate with that formula. So it will be good to improve the recipe or to change it altogether. Christ performed most of his healing instantaneously by himself, often just through using his voice. So if you are strong in yourself you will not need anyone to help you. But if you always work alone without joining a group you may miss something. The value of belonging to a large organization such as, for example, the National Federation of Spiritual Healers,* is that of being linked to a store of knowledge. So it is good to join a healing organization and to meet other healers in order to exchange ideas and to learn and develop

*The National Federation of Spiritual Healers, Old Manor Farm Studio, Church St, Sunbury-on-Thames, runs a number of courses for those wishing to learn and to qualify as healers.

the finer points of the art. There is another point. If you always practise individually without ever joining and losing yourself in a group there is a danger that you will produce a huge ego. Alternatively, if you only work in groups and never do any work on your own you may lose your ego to an extent that you will be useless. If you have no sense of yourself you cannot pull yourself, pull your atoms together, you will be spread all over the universe. You have to have a sense of identity to be able to form somewhere. The ego is there as a standard of reference encapsulating the survival instinct. As you space out more, ironically you will need a bigger ego with which to earth. The more you want to space out the more your system will have to establish *you*. With the 'I' we can space out and have something to return to. The 'I' is like an island in the consciousness. But often this island grows into a bastille which we are unable to control, it becomes a monument to inner needs and desires. We have to establish a true identification of self, the spiritual 'I AM', which resounds in the heart, the source of our being, the source of our rhythm and our beat.

More information on working in a group is given in Appendix II.

Protection

This means surrounding ourselves and our patients with a positive shield of energy so that no unwanted thought forms or entities can invade our space. It means closing down the chakras so that negative forces cannot bother us. All of us have the potential to project a cloak of many colours round us, a radiant cloak of light. But really the greatest protection of all is our ability to radiate strong energies from our bodies. If we are a loving generous person with no tension in our body, our radiance can be so strong that we will automatically enjoy an armour of protective energy enveloping us. Some individuals have the notion that we should never protect ourselves, but should go round as open as possible. This is an idealistic way of looking at things and generally we find such attitudes in people who are either just starting in the work or who have particularly strong energy-fields. Certainly this ideal state is one we should be aiming towards: one in which everyone is able to open their chakras and exchange energies liberally – the aura and the heart thrive, as we know, on exchanging energies with everything. Perhaps one day it will be possible for us to go round open all the time, yet these days it is not practical for most of us. Of course if we live in a protected environment we never need to close. Providing we are always well, providing we have strong energies, we can certainly go round open. If we walk down a crowded city street or travel on a London underground train we will do a lot of cleansing, which is excellent providing we have systems which can purify themselves. The trouble is that some of us cannot purify ourselves automatically. Some of us become ill or gather so much tension that we come out in allergies, or find that we are unable to earth properly. So be aware that if you sometimes feel low and depressed, or if your health is not good, then it is better to put some form of protection round you.

There are many ways of doing this. Breathing around the aura is one of the most protective exercises we can do. Or we can breathe a pyramid around us and cover it with gold – we can reach the golden dimensions by breathing in gold continually. We can use white light as a protection: a beam of energy. You can think of yourself being surrounded by a column of light. Some people when they are working concentrate on making a column of light in their room so that heavy negative energies are unable to get through.

Colour Healing and How to Project It

Each ray of colour has its guardian angel, so remember that we can never be instrumental in any form of colour healing without the angel participating as an integral part of the weave. There are various ways of exerting colour. We can use the rays themselves as tools, as something separate from ourselves. We can take a figure of a man to represent our patient and with lamps or slides shine upon him the relevant rays. We can use a colour table upon which we place the

116

names of our patients in the appropriate section. If our patient, for example, needs red we will put him in the red section and so on. We can have a room which may be illuminated in the required hue. We can programme crystals. We can project mentally an image of our patient on the wall and shower him with colour. We can learn, either by using our pendulum or directly with our intuition, that our patient needs a particular colour – let us say green – and we can sit there and concentrate on conducting green and letting it flow to the patient. But whatever the colour we should never project it until either the pendulum or our intuition informs us, or the colour somehow manifests in our minds. If there is any doubt it is always preferable to use white light, which contains the whole spectrum.

There is another way: to use our own body as a colour instrument. If we link our higher selves to the angels of colour this will produce the possibility of our being an instrument, a vessel, which will bring through the correct colour for the patient without our doing anything. This will not be a case of conscious projection but of linking with the highest which can flow through and radiate the vibration to the patient. We become the vibration rather than using our will to project it consciously. Remember that, through tuning into the highest realms, our possibilities are unlimited, by tuning into particular colours we limit our scope.

Whatever technique we practise we always have to raise our energies and change our brainwaves in the usual fashion. People like to work in different ways. Through exercising the highest levels we ourselves become the colour instrument while, by means of mental or physical projection, we apply the rays as something separate. So be aware that there is a difference between projecting a colour and going through to yourself. In the latter case you feel the vibration, you become it and, by becoming part of it, you will resonate at that level and with attunement your patient will pick up that resonance.

It is a good idea to give your patients visualization exercises which will incorporate colour through envisaging nature. For example, you can take them for a walk in the country. You can get them to think of a lovely sunny day as you start off. You walk through a green meadow full of spring flowers, you can go through a wood if you like, bring in the blue of water and sky, a few white clouds. Looking at flowers, water and sky, whether mentally or physically, is healing, so is everything to do with the air. Helping people to imagine such things will take them to the higher realms and assist them to change their minds.

6

Physical and Psychic
Environmental Influences

Fear and the distress, the tension it engenders are factors
which underlie all illness and should be understood.

In primitive society fear was a fact of life. In other words,
it was an essential measure for survival. It triggered off the
mechanism that generated the power to deal with danger
which, in those days, was almost always tangible. In order
to live you either had to fight the peril or to run away from
it. Nowadays so many of the things that threaten us are
intangible, difficult to fight physically or psychically, or even
to run away from. In any case, most of us are too unfit to
do either. Nevertheless, whenever we are confronted with
anything menacing, our primeval instinct still comes up with
the necessary power to deal with it and when we do not use
this power either for running away or for fighting but control
ourselves in a 'civilized' manner, we build up a great deal of
pressure which becomes difficult to release.

So fear is a primordial instinct necessary for evolution,
which creates a state of tension. Tension is always associated
with our sense of separateness. We perceive a threat to our
individuality and so fear arises: albeit fear of pain, fear of
isolation, fear of the unknown or the ultimate fear of death.
This is why self-exploration is important. Through meditation and contemplation we may recognize what it is we
are fearing, what it is that is hampering our thought process.
Frédéric Lionel, the French mystic and teacher, speaks about
this succinctly. By searching diligently we will perceive that
the seed of fear lies in the phenomenon of opposites, of
duality. Being engaged in a dual world we oppose the two

119

poles and fear arises. To overcome fear we have to overcome duality, we have to reach the truth beyond separation. We have to go beyond the false pretence that 'my interest is contrary to yours' that 'I can escape fear by asserting my power'. Fusion on every level is necessary. We see it, for example, in sexual union. Two people united in one soul; in total integration of their essential beings they forget themselves. There is total relinquishment, one with the other and fusion is manifested. We return again to the emblem of Asklepios: the snake winding up the staff; the reconciliation of opposites; man's most holy goal. When we fall from this state of harmony and become perturbed our survival mechanism comes into play, ready for fight or flight, and our solar plexus becomes overcharged. This applies equally when we have tantrums or endure distressing circumstances. When we hate other people, our work and our families, when we feel inferior or superior, when we create situations from which we want to escape, we will have problems with the solar plexus which will resound in the heart and the third eye. Our balance will be disturbed and we may have duodenal problems, become dizzy, break out in sweats and allergies and even, ultimately, become subject to heart attacks.

The minute we are afraid of something our energies stop projecting, they stop radiating and turn back in on themselves. When problems start at a young age they may manifest increasingly at puberty. In other words when a chakra system opens prematurely through shock or accident, the child may suffer emotional disturbances and in adolescence turn to drugs, alcohol or smoking to dull the pain. Then if his diet is inadequate or his natural breathing and the amount of exercise he takes is not enough to clear his system, a point of stagnation may be reached where old memories will be revived — patterns which will repeat the weaknesses set up in early life. These flaws may increase under stress so that the situation may worsen and the etheric grows coarse, thereby attracting negativity. Indeed there is always the danger to any of us that if we get into a state of exhaustion, if we are drained, we will attract negativity to ourselves which can manifest in various ways, one of them being depression.

Sometimes the childhood years of pain can be forgotten as a person matures. Perhaps he marries happily and everything starts to flow beautifully until something happens to make life difficult again and the flaws and patterns surface once more – such memories can trigger off all kinds of illness.

Stress, as we have seen, affects all the organs of the body. For one thing it produces too much cortisone so that the immune system goes down. For another the release mechanism seizes up so that the excretory areas cannot function well which constitutes a serious handicap, often bringing a whole change of outlook: depression and fatigue. Vibrations of hate and fear can produce glandular changes and biochemical results which can be estimated in a laboratory.

We could say that we become trapped in a vicious circle. When we are tired, tense and worried, we dissipate energy, we become drained and draw to us negative energies which make us more depressed. In order to survive our energies tune into the heavier particles which form a wall of protection through which pain cannot be felt so acutely. The body, meanwhile, needing to exert more energy to live, begins to turn to quick methods of stimulation, for example smoking, drinking and strong coffee. The toxic effect of these will filter through into the etheric and the two systems will break down so that we are plunged further down into depression, or what is sometimes called the dark night of the soul.

We know that if a healer is under stress and suffering from depression and he turns to smoking and/or drinking the healing will cleanse him. But if his energies do not align well and he continues to be depressed and give healing, his system will eventually collapse and illness will ensue. A healer may continue to work even if he is ill, he may pass strong charges through weakened circuits, but this might lead him to an early death. It is true that most healers find it easier to give healing to several people rather than spend the equivalent time in sorting out themselves. Like all human beings they have a tendency to ignore their own weaknesses and not see themselves as others do. If a healer has health problems he needs to look at his own stress and he probably needs to go to another healer to be helped physically and mentally. In other words, perhaps he needs to practise what he preaches.

Sensitivity to Environment

As we become more sensitive, as we progress on etheric levels, we may experience difficulties. For example, primitive man was far more aware than most of us of changes in the weather. He knew if bad weather, hurricanes or earthquakes were approaching. This means that as we grow more sensitive we, too, may react more to atmospheric pressure. As the barometer falls our spirits may follow suit or we may start to stiffen. Aches and pains may mean that our environment is affecting us; this can build up tension at the back of the neck and round the shoulders. Eating seaweed and mussels can help but quite often we need to look carefully at our environment. We can, sometimes, grow out of districts. If we are strong we can cope with, even cleanse, any area, but if for any reason we do not have that kind of strength we may be better off elsewhere. Again we can grow out of people and become allergic to their energies.

There are so many signals we can pick up. We can become like wireless transmitters and this has its problems. There are so many wars, so much pollution on every level. If we are sensitive, every time we listen to the news can be a shock to the system and the shock may keep the chakras open too long. We must make sure that we purify the body often; even so, there may always be something constantly wrong with us which does not originate from ourselves but which we pick up from other people or the environment. Some healers absorb pain from their patients, sometimes they absorb it from the atmosphere. All of us need a sense of humour and detachment and then with objectivity we can sort out and deal with these things.

Every day we are bombarded with electro-magnetic stresses which are alien to our systems. Radio, micro-waves, telegraph signals and telephone calls expose body, brain and organs to stress. Albert Roy Davis and Walter C. Rawls in their book, *Rainbow in Your Hands*, claim that when a number of telephones were checked in the United States it was discovered that they radiated positive (unbeneficial) energy of a strength to penetrate the skull into the brain. Electric shavers produce alternating currents of electro-magnetic energy that also pass into the head and so do electric toothbrushes. Even television is potentially dangerous, especially coloured sets, when we are exposed to them for too long. One of the rays is similar to X-ray which is known to be damaging in large quantities. Thousands of miles of high-voltage cables cross the country owing to the national electric-grid system. It is now known that through a process known as corona – which produces ozone, a poisonous gas which can be harmful to animals and plants – these high-voltage transmission lines can cause electrical breakdown of the air in the immediate vicinity of the wires. More controversial are the electro-magnetic fields which the wires create. Some scientists claim that these can affect living organisms. The results can be a speeding up or a slowing down of responses, stunted growth or development of tumours.

Thoughtforms

It is a fact that, on one level, we are surrounded by evil. We are here to purify and transform all the negativity that man has put out into the atmosphere through his destructive thoughts. One of the basic essentials of healing is to be able to dissolve thoughtforms: in other words to be able to clear peoples' minds.

Before going further it may be helpful to look into the nature of good and evil. We could say that our aim is to be beyond all good, beyond all evil, but until such a time as we have overcome duality we will be bound by these laws. We could say again that evil is the pollution we have caused through our mistakes. It is those energies which have darkened, become coarse, and, being unable to rise to higher levels, attract others to them, pulling them down to their levels. The psychiatrist Dr Arthur Guirdham, who has made a study* of psychic forces and evil as a cause of disease, takes this further. Good and evil can be regarded either as ethical concepts or they can be experienced as radiating

---

Obsession by Arthur Guirdham, published by Neville Spearman, London 1972.

123

forces, palpable vibrations like sound, light and heat: vibratory emanations of immense power and scope. It is the nature of these forces, as Dr Guirdham points out, that has exercised all organized religions in the past (just as the eternal conflict between them is the basis of all modern crime and adventure stories). In these days the problem has been resolved by many scientists (including many psychiatrists), by the simple process of denying their existence. Evil has been replaced by anti-social behaviour and maladjustment. This, Dr Guirdham observes, sounds well enough in theory but too many exponents of materialist psychiatry would regard as anti-social anything not answering to immediate herd-requirements. In other words creative art and religious experience would easily be classified as anti-social.

Part of our system, then, is to oppose things that can affect us in a negative way whether they be bacteria or thoughtforms. Negative thoughts cause coarse textures to form in the aura. We can imagine them looking a bit like the heavy weave of sackcloth. Let us suppose that we release a negative or an evil thought. By a reverse mechanism it deepens the darkness in our hearts and reverberates internally in the nervous and glandular system. A greater concentration of evil can impregnate the air, polluting the atmosphere, contaminating the place and having palpable effects on all those exposed to it. The external and ubiquitous effects of hate and other negative emotions in the atmosphere are universal and, in the view of Dr Guirdham, their destructive power is incalculable. The energy of every evil thought is disseminated through the universe, harming everyone.

This can affect us in two ways. Either it can lodge in a discarnate being or it can pollute people or places through manifesting as thoughtforms. There are so many thoughts around us in the ether, so many ideas in people's minds and many of them ugly. These can have a debilitating effect, especially in crowded cities, and we need to get away regularly to open parks and spaces, the countryside and the sea.

First, though, it is important to understand the nature of thoughtforms and to know the difference between these and entities. Thoughts are things which take shape in the ether.

124

Sometimes what we take to be a ghost is a very strong thoughtform which has impressed itself upon the ether. Perhaps we are in a house and we see something or someone passing a few inches higher or lower than ground level, doing exactly the same thing every time we see them. This is likely to be an impression rather than an entity. It does not see us, nor in any way is it involved with us. What we are doing is watching a film. It is possible to get rid of these impressions by rubbing them out etherically or we can breathe into them, disintegrate their forms by dancing or chanting, but, if the impression is deep, it may keep recurring until it wears out.

Everything that has manifested on this planet started as a thoughtform, an impression on the ether. The ancient Egyptians and the Druids used to create huge thoughtforms by exerting the energies from trees and stones; they took these thoughtforms with them into battle to fight the enemy. Thoughtforms attack by unwinding themselves and projecting into the aura of the person under assault. When a negative thought is directed to us it moves – like all vibrations – in waves. Frustration, hate, bitterness, all these can wind up huge coils of tension inside the invaded subject.

Yet we we must remember that what one is receiving is energy and any energy is capable of being converted. So if a thoughtform arrives within range of our aura we may be able to transform it. Some people can transmute attacks with the outer edge of their aura so that, when the thoughtform hits it, it is either deflected or dissolved. But if the outer edge is weak the thoughtform may penetrate the auric space. Even so, radiations from the hundreds of tiny surface chakras can still take and dissolve it. But people who are low in energy for any reason, who have little power in their electrical circuits, will be obliged to contract their auras for protection, since subconsciously they will be afraid of any approaching negativity. This forms a grey wall around them and often destructive thoughts coming in will hit this and either hang about the fringe or be absorbed into the earth. People with strong circuits have a reflecting mechanism in their chakras and everything that is sent to them will be bounced back and returned to sender, although not necessarily transmuted.

Imagine, then, that a negative thought is thrown at you

and you are conscious of it being there. You can transform it and send back love. Love is such a powerful force that if you can do this often enough a negative person will be able to release his frustration and clear the aura around him. If a person consciously uses his rational left-brain to try to affect another this will be felt in his target's solar plexus which should be able to receive the energy and transmute it. If the solar plexus is already overcharged with negativity the energy, instead of transmuting, can only add to what is already there. Sometimes destructive thoughts can be projected unconsciously by the right side of the brain in which case the target, suddenly for no apparent reason, may find himself visited with a headache. It may be helpful to know that left-brain negativity can be dissolved by the sun, while adversity from the right hemisphere of the brain may be broken down by rays from the moon. Water, sea and the healing blue of the sky also disperse thoughtforms.

So if a negative thought flows into your consciousness you can transmute it creatively. You can open up the energy-fields over the head or make the radiations in the feet stronger and, with your own thoughts, re-shape the projection. See it as a water-lily, form it into a spotless crystal. It is good to pray for the person who is conducting negativity: prayer always links us with the highest and brings down energy. When hands are radiating well they too will dissolve thought-forms. Sometimes we find that we move our hands about, gesticulating, without knowing why we are doing it.

Sometimes individuals create thoughtforms out of fear or lack of confidence. 'I can't do this; I am not worthy of doing that.' If such thoughts get too big they can take people over: thus they are possessed by themselves. It is possible to exorcise such possession by changing the thought patterns.

Possession

When looking at the subject of possession we must remember that, as usual, there are two aspects to the phenomenon: good and bad. For thousands of years possession has been deliberately induced to give human beings direct experience of a deity, or holy spirit, through becoming its living vessel, thus enabling humans to act as a channel of communication between the gods and their worshippers. When a person is seen to be possessed he loses control; his personality seems obliterated, he is not able to think for himself and something impinges on his mind. We can, in fact, be possessed by different things – we have seen that our own negativity can possess us. But, basically, we can either be possessed by a negative thoughtform or an external entity. Of course there are good spirits and bad; angels, after all, are entities or discarnate beings. Some spirits are decidedly bad and we do have to be careful. We may require the backing and support of professionals to deal with them. Some entities have a need that has never been sorted out. One girl, for example, had terrible trouble with her father who had died. He desperately wanted a requiem mass and he was prepared to invade the house and everyone in it with his misery, to ruin their lives, in order to get it. Again some entities invade people for their own gratification, this level of entity is generally in pursuit of some kind of sexual experience.

Dr Sargant who witnessed many ritual ceremonies for the casting out of spirits in Africa, Haiti, Brazil and Trinidad, observed that the primitive methods of curing the sick, by evacuating undesirable entities, followed the same sort of patterns as modern drug treatments. States of excitement were induced leading to tremendous emotional and muscular discharge which ended in almost total collapse. In Africa, where most illness, unless seen to be obviously organic, is traditionally held to be caused by spirit possession, the treatment is a ceremonial drumming out of the demons. The patients move round and round in a circle until they fall into the all-important trance and writhe, twitching and jerking, on the ground. Sometimes, during the trance the ancestral spirits will communicate through the patients, revealing much useful information as to the nature of the illness. Later, during a ceremony which Sargant found particularly impressive, they speak through the witch-doctor himself. The ancestral spirits, giving their interpretation of the causes of illness, seemed to him far more effective than modern psychoanalysis. Some of the ceremonies involved fumigation rather than drumming and dancing. The devils were smoked out. A cloth was placed over the patient's head so that he was obliged to breathe in the heavy fumes emitted from a heap of burning herbs on a brazier.

The Catholic Church has never denied the existence of the devil, nor possession by evil spirits. One of Christ's best-known healings is the casting out of evil spirits to the swine. Ritual exorcism used to hold a special place in Christianity. Yet since 1664 no clergyman of the Church of England has been allowed to cast out devils and nowadays any Roman Catholic priest requires a special licence to practise exorcism. Lately the Church has made efforts to keep up with the times. The devil, it is felt, is not part of modern life. Possession tests credulity and there has been a gradual playing down of the mysterious or supernatural elements so that, when one of the basic theology texts used at the Jesuit's Gregorian University in Rome, was revised, the section on angels and demons was omitted from the new edition – which is ironic considering the increase of interest in magic and the occult.

Entities, nevertheless, do exist and they can take over certain individuals so we should know something about them. Some are lost souls roaming the earth, some are holding on to earth levels, too negative and heavy to move higher. In order to exorcise and transform such beings, attention should be paid to the whole vehicle of the possessed person. The physical body should be strengthened and correctly nourished. To make the individual secure it is a good idea to start by cleaning and purifying his house, dusting and spring cleaning it. But some people feel safer with their own vibrations scattered about and sometimes a spring cleaning can bring a crisis of insecurity – when dealing with entities it is best never to go to extremes. Make the whole atmosphere as pure as possible. Purify the environment and the mind by reading good literature and surrounding the place with candles, incense and spiritual colours.

Really the greatest ally when dealing with entities is the left-brain. You have to avoid imagination and you have to avoid fear. Fear makes a person easy to take over. Lilla has a story of a very kind person, living in a haunted house, who kept having a frightful apparition appear at the foot of her bed. 'Oh hallo dear, there you are again', she would say. 'I'm off to sleep now, if you want you can go away or you can stay there, it's quite all right.'

The apparition would make horrid growling noises. 'That's all right dear,' the woman would say, 'make as many of those as you like, I don't mind. You can do a little dance, too, it's all right by me.' This went on for weeks and every night the woman would say, 'Blessings on you! Good night, I'm off to sleep now.' After three months the apparition started to change and one day the most beautiful man appeared and thanked her very much and went away. The story is told here basically to illustrate the quality of love, strength and optimism that is required for dealing with negative forces. It is essential never to allow fear to intrude.

Really, it is not wise to try to fight an entity by yourself; it is far more sensible to work with a group or to call in the help of a professional exorcist. Nevertheless, if you are alone and obliged to deal with a negative force wherever possible use candles, holy oils and holy water to help you. It cannot be reiterated too often: it is essential that you eliminate fear. If you light a candle with shaking hands and you try to put incense round the room while you are trembling with fright, you will not have enough energy going through to the subconscious levels to produce the necessary powers to deal with the force. This is because fear has a heavy vibration (and also a particular smell) and if you do anything when you are frightened, even if it is making a sign of the cross, it cannot be potent. Behind any successful exorcism there has to be power. Take the example of prayer. If you just vaguely mutter some words with your heart and mind elsewhere, the prayer will not be active. Remember that behind anything, behind lighting a candle, placing a vase of flowers, saying a prayer, is the attention with which you do it. Even if you call upon God, Christ, the archangels or saints to help you, you can only call upon them with the energy you are generating at the time. It is when you have unbounded confidence, enthusiasm and fire that things will happen.

You might even try having a conversation with the entity. Remember that entities do not need to be wicked, they may just be miserable. After all, any sort of darkness is really unhappiness of some sort. If talking does not help, and incense and candles have not worked, then you might try using a practical approach and subject the entity to a barrage of questions. How long have you been doing it? How many years? Use geometrical shapes: project circles and crosses. Remember that negative entities can fill the room and every time you breathe in you can absorb this negativity into yourself. So you must consciously draw in light. You can do this by sucking it down through the head and sending it out through the feet in a continuous flow. You can imagine the cleansing vibration of gold pouring through the body and out through the feet. You can project a sacred sound at the entity like Om, use other sacred chants, you can whip up a lot of energy by dancing. If you move in circles and use the hands you can produce a strong energy and a good momentum. So remember, whenever you have to fight, your success will depend on the amount of energy you can raise. So first and foremost when dealing with entities avoid fear. Ask for help from the highest levels, from the saints and angels. Imagine the sword of truth, put a gold protective crown on your head, think of yourself as a knight shielded with an armour of light. Make golden crosses and circles on the chakras.

Like all negativity, entities have to be released from the body through the pores and the bowels. This is one of the reasons why fear has to be abolished. Fear causes tension and tension inhibits the release mechanism. Medieval exorcism often involved crude and cruel cleansing techniques which must have made the possessed person even more terrified. Since the devil was associated with the bowels many ritualistic exorcisms included the enforced insertion of enemas. Some of the best ways to release are through deep breathing and laughter and, as we have seen from the traditional ceremonies, dancing and movement.

Father Francis MacNutt, who is an expert on exorcism, says the ceremony should end successfully in coughing and retching as the entity is ejected. Prayer must follow in order to fill the person in question with God's love and grace. It is essential, he says, that the vacuum caused by the ejection

130

of the entity be filled by the presence of Jesus and the person should be taught to break his habitual behaviour patterns that have led him to demonic infestation, some kind of spiritual discipline being substituted to combat his weakness and compete with the spirits of envy, resentment and so on.

Negative entities dislike purity. They dislike pure bodies and pure minds. So every time a negative thought enters the consciousness supplant it with a beautiful one. They dislike spiritual company, healers and churches. So if we constantly try to raise the levels the entity will generally depart. We can try using holy symbols or prayers designed to be applied in an emergency. Such is the prayer known as St Patrick's breastplate:

Christ be with me; Christ be within me,
Christ before me; Christ behind me,
Christ on my right hand; Christ on my left hand.
Christ above me; Christ beneath me,
Christ round about me.

Obsession often marches with possession. When a person becomes obsessed to the point of illness it is usually a protective reflex because they have been overwhelmed, possessed by a sensation of evil. They may become obsessed with the need to clean and purify themselves, obsessed with certain kinds of dreams, obsessed with their negativity or with the belief that others are trying to harm them.

The Nature of Disease

We have seen that ancient civilizations (together with many peoples still retaining their traditional beliefs and customs) maintained that disease was caused by the invasion of evil spirits. The idea that the genesis of disease involves the power of evil would be regarded today as repugnant, as superstitious nonsense. Yet this is precisely what, in some cases, could be proposed. Dr Guirdham cites the case of virus infections. A certain number will ultimately be identified as being due to particular organisms, or the poisons they

131

secrete, but, excluding these, there is an enormous number of cases diagnosed as virus infections for no other reason than that the laboratory can discover nothing to account for their existence. These infections are some of the greatest mysteries of modern medicine and are characterized by great enfeeblement and an intense feeling of malaise. The patient becomes dispirited, hopeless, often considerably depressed, without capacity to fight back, and often the only clinical sign is a mild temperature perhaps in the evenings. Dr Guirdham observes that these symptoms of virus infection correspond largely to those presented by victims of malign forces in what are regarded as the more primitive communities: total enfeeblement, physical symptoms of comparative triviality, listlessness, depression and a mysterious cause.

There is nothing new either in suggesting that the roots of many of our problems can be traced back to a period of our lives, which to all intent and purpose appears to have been forgotten. Dr Guirdham, again, has found that many problems can be traced back to the earliest years of childhood and sometimes beyond to past lives. It may take decades for disturbances that were created in an earlier life to come to the intensity of physical manifestation we recognize as illness. One way of dealing with these deep-seated traumas is regression, which can be a useful tool for allaying embedded fears.

Every year the medical world finds more medicines to counteract illness and infection, yet it is ultimately up to us to take our disease into our own hands and deal with it. How often do we sit back and rely on antibiotics and other drugs? Modern medicine means that we accept disease and treat the symptoms without trying to reach an understanding of how it is affecting us on deeper levels. We blame doctors for treating the symptoms but, in many respects, we do the same. Until we are able to trace the illnesses back to the roots, even if necessary back to birth and beyond, there will never be a complete cure for many people.

Really, disease should not exist at all. If our vitality is strong and flowing freely we should, in theory, never be attacked by any serious illness. It is possible to stay healthy. But whenever a debilitated person works with or even meets others who are unfit, whether etherically or physically, disease will spread.

So many of us cause our problems through ambition. We strive to reach the top (and healers and psychics are just as vulnerable in this as anyone else) and sometimes set ourselves impossible goals which we cannot achieve and so we become acutely anxious. We must accept then that we cause our illnesses and our problems ourselves. Thanks to freedom of choice we have the possibility of taking initiatives. If these lead to actions that oppose the laws of harmony then we violate our nature. Edgar Cayce observed (together with the orthodox Church in those early centuries) that all illness comes from sin whether of mind, body or soul. This is not a moralistic use of the word but the use of the word 'sin' to mean a violation of a law. For the sake of clarification let us say that sin is negativity which produces psychological disturbances – fears, anxieties, tensions and so on. If we take something simple like someone always telling lies, it means that he has to remember which lies he has told to whom and for this he is constantly using up energy. Then to maintain this false world he has to continue fabricating it so that not only does he have to remember what lies he has told in the past, he has to continue them and if he is unable to remember everything this can create awkward situations and tension which may eventually manifest as disease. Alternatively, we could take a man who is married and at the same time having an affair with another woman. This puts extra pressure on him because he has to be two-sided. He needs all that extra energy in order to do something here with his wife and then go off and do something there with his friend. He leads a dual life which again creates tensions and difficulties and may eventually manifest in illness.

We can expand this by saying that it is often guilt that ruins a person's health. Much illness is caused by people regretting their actions, feeling that they should not have acted in such and such a way in the past, that they should somehow be entirely different: non-aggressive perhaps, always sweet and uncomplaining whatever happens. They are riddled with hidden frustrations they are unable to release. We must accept ourselves as we really are. We return again to the fundamental instruction of the temples: self-exploration so that we may know ourselves.

So many of us have a lot of faults. We go through life with bad habits of which we know very little. Often we present a face to the world which is beautifully painted and cared for, while inside we are disintegrating. To pretend that everything is all right when the opposite is true leads to suppression and when we suppress things we block our flow of energy and prevent it from functioning properly. It is the hidden things in the mind that are the inhibiting factors of life. Everything we repress will be a source of disease.

If we are aware and can accept that our illness comes from a previous disharmonious origin, if we can accept that we ourselves have caused our illness by our behaviour, whether in this or in past lives, health may be restored. We have first to accept our condition and then ask why: What is the message for me? Is it fear of not being able to achieve something? Is it uneasiness which may lead to a flight into something different? In these days we must not succumb or react to our primordial instinct of fight or flight. We must look carefully and learn. Sometimes a lesson has to be learnt from the illness and until this happens it will be impossible to heal. So we must try to decipher the message and learn the lesson the disease is teaching us.

The root of any disease lies dormant in negative etheric patterns until such time as emotional or mental pressures create the possibility for the etheric to manifest its disturbed energy in the physical body. Let us take the example of cancer. The disease begins on etheric levels with unhappiness and tension gathering and being unable to release naturally, either through excretion or exhalation. Inadequate diet, over-indulgence and inability to relax will also help the disease to manifest. We could say that cancer is the misalignment of energy patterns due to stresses which cannot be dealt with at various stages of development and in consequence have upset the energy-fields. Cancer is a condition which feeds particularly on rotten conditions of mind and body. Where there is no waste there will be no cancer. But imbalance in a cell may prevent it from maturing and functioning correctly so that it begins to accumulate poison and thrive on waste materials. When a cell multiplies prematurely it becomes disorganized – its reaction is not unlike that of a two-year-old child who, unable to cope with its environment, retires into its shell for protection – the result being that the necessary energy exchanges are impaired. Energies should radiate outwards, meet others and exchange. With disease they double back and become self-centred. We can see this reflected in ill people who become self-obsessed and egocentric. Some people when they fall ill are unable to give anything to anybody. It is actually the act of taking, of gathering energy and not giving or releasing it, that is making them ill. When we find someone who is unable to share, something is wrong. In order for the cancerous tumour to be dissolved the body needs to bring about a dramatic change. Growths are generally a sign of some malfunction of the mind, some kind of attitude to life; it could even be a wish to leave the world and destroy the self. Sometimes they mean that we are living with people who are eating up all our energies so that we are constantly dissipating our vitality. It is in any case essential to bring the information to the surface so that the patient can release his fear, anxiety and anger, that is so deeply embedded.

We know that by working on the etheric body spiritual healers can neutralize any disease by realigning the energies and restoring them to harmony so as to unleash the body's natural curative ability. It is of course difficult to help someone to health if he has been all wrong since the age of two and has continued to be all wrong for the following fifty years. Certainly not everyone gets healed. A healer may be fully experienced, he may radiate a huge energy and be excellent with specific types of illness; however, he is still dependent on his patient. If a person erects a barrier, a wall of fear, no matter how powerful the energies of the healer may be he will be unlikely to break through. Some people will not get better simply because their time has come to die. When people have finished their mission on earth there is nothing a healer can do to stop them from dying. Indeed it is sometimes the attitude to death that has to be healed. Sometimes the dying is the healing. Aside from this some

135

people will not get better because it is their karma to live through the illness and learn from it. If an illness fails to respond either to orthodox treatment or to healing, we can presume that it is karmic. If there is karma to be paid, or there are lessons to be learnt, the patient may become calmer and happier, he may or may not be helped to bear his illness better, but the illness will not be removed.

The idea of karma is that of cause and effect. Everything that we do leaves a trace which cannot be wiped off. In this way the past affects the present, every action, every thought has final consequences which cannot be changed. No one can get rid of the past. Everything negative that we do will reverberate within us and eventually affect us. If we dissipate our powers, if we exploit others, appropriate energy and abuse it, this will have an accumulative obligation and will have to be paid for in this life or a future one. In such cases we gather liabilities to the point of saturation, until we are unable to borrow any more, and then we start to repay. We have to be aware that, as we find our spiritual path and begin to dissolve the coarse particles in our aura the paying of karma will accelerate. To put it another way, as our auric space becomes cleansed it causes our karma to manifest in such a way that it often seems as though our lives are falling apart. So we should never wonder why our lives appear to become worse as we try to become better. Repaying karmic debts can certainly be an unhappy experience and some people, not realizing what is going on, become bitter. So often there is a reaction: 'Here I am trying to mend my ways and help others to lead a good life: why am I suffering?' So if we find our path we should not complain or be frustrated by the suffering and challenges we meet along the way; we should settle down, accept them and learn our lessons.

The higher self will always want to repay karma in any way it can. Every healer will want to repay and some years of a healer's life may seem particularly painful and difficult as he does so. If he abuses his body he may have frustrations which he will suffer to even the score. Some healers take on another person's illness to free them from their karma and past mistakes. The highest aspect of any human being feels

136

responsible for his own mistakes and will never feel free until he has repaid his debts.

If you heal a person and he fails to pay you, thank you, or become more generous in some way, that person will accrue a karmic debt, either to you or to the whole of humanity for the rest of his life. There always has to be an exchange of some sort and some people do need information while receiving healing: they should be aware that if they receive healing yet give nothing back they will be producing encumbrances for themselves. The temples allowed people to give what they could: food perhaps, jewellery, livestock, children. We always have to give and to take according to the rhythm of life. Recovery can be complete only through generosity. If your patients never show generosity to you, it is you who is at fault. Christ touched people's hearts, he opened them so that they became giving and understanding. A few healers charge exorbitant fees. It might be argued that they are freeing their patients from the karmic debts that come into operation after each healing but, in taking too much, the healer may himself incur a debt.

We can repay karma by taking upon ourselves difficult lives and situations which cause illness. But usually illness is a result of not listening to our inner voice, of trying to change life rather than ourselves. If we do not accept our illness, if we fight it and go against that which, in the light of evolution, we may need to learn, instead of burning off karma we might cause more. Karma is not just what we have done in the past, it is what we are doing now. Let us pause and reflect for a moment. What is your mind doing at this minute? How are your vibrations *now*?

We have to examine ourselves carefully, look at our reasons for coming down to earth in the first place and for our suffering. All this must be explored and no amount of pills will give us the answer. Certainly pills will help the physical body to recover from an illness but the root of the disturbance will survive, leading to further complications in later life.

Life is movement and movement is life. For evolution there has to be duality. In other words, in order for awareness to grow there has to be someone who is aware of something.

137

We are the witnesses and the actors on the stage of the world and the play can only go on thanks to us. The whole of our past, up to this moment, is a film; the whole of the future is also a projected film which relies on the past. Thus we are only in the present for a fraction of time. All the world is a stage and we re-enact certain roles over and over again. The film comes round and round until we realize the part we have chosen and can fathom what it is we have to learn. And in this film it is the mind and the vibrations which are important. We are what the mind is: what our vibrations are. In Egypt if you had trouble with your role, trouble, let us say, with your mother, a play would be made out of it. You would have to act yourself as the child, then you would have to act the part of the mother and in this way you would see things from a different point of view. You would be seeing the play from your mother's angle.

Every time we come down we have to face something new, some new challenge. We could say that the world is a laboratory in which we sit the test of daily existence. It will not be the experience that is important so much as the vibrations and the rays we establish. To pass the test we must stabilize the appropriate rays.

In this world we lack the security we long for. Ironically, nothing on earth is certain apart from our death. If only we could come to terms with death we would be able to enjoy our lives better. We have made such giants out of illness and death. Yet death is not the end, it is but a transition. Facing death was one of the initiatory rites. You lay in a tomb and remained in darkness for forty hours and if you could overcome your trials you were accepted into the inner circle. Illness and death are both transitions, they are crossings. Illness is usually for leading us to a more spiritual state so that we can make a new beginning. It is in this sense nothing but an initiation. Ancient civilizations had the equivalent of midwives to help the dying pass over. Unfortunately, in our modern world we refuse to face up to death and usually go unprepared. One of the most important jobs of any healing – including self-healing – is to prepare ourselves and our patients for death. The Church has discouraged people from searching into the mysteries, has denied all personal knowledge of the supernatural, yet it does not really play a part in helping people to understand or cope with these things. Many priests and clergymen are themselves afraid of death – together with being apprehensive, or dismissive of, healing, wary of ghosts and possession and suspicious of psychic gifts.

By reconciling ourselves to that great restorative process we can detach ourselves more easily from the body and so identify with the spirit. Healing is not just helping people to live, it is helping people to cross over. Providing we are not too attached to our bodies and this earthly plane, the crossing can be superb. Many will find the end beautiful: the ultimate liberation: the getting away from it all. It is simply a speeding up and can bring with it a marvellous sense of light and youth and happiness. You can see this sometimes reflected in a dying person's face: the complete tranquillity. Sometimes people, as they approach death, see beautiful things, crystal structures, buildings, cities of light. Some will see the film of their life unfolding. Often friends come to help. Many people as they grow older have more friends 'upstairs' than here on earth. Dying can and should be a beautiful experience, rather like a huge party – after all we are only going back home. Yet so often our deaths are hampered by our last thoughts, our needs at the point of going. Our friends and our guides may try to get through and we may not be able to reach out. Sometimes, as in the case of accidents, people may be projected very quickly out of the body and find it difficult to accept they are on a different dimension. They are so attached to their bodies and their friends that they do not want to leave the earth. They become disoriented and the guides are unable to make contact.

Our last thought before death is important. Just as the last thought that we take into meditation will establish the mood of the meditation so the last thought before we die will establish the realms we will be able to contact after death. If our mind is occupied with the needs we have created during our life these will bog us down. If we long for the security of a nice house in which to live, or we desire to eat and drink a great deal and have sex, these needs will continue until eventually the urges die. We will have to go through

139

them again and again until we can go beyond. If we cannot let go of our ideas we will be drawn back to them again and again. So let us be aware of the importance of our last thoughts: the last thought before going to sleep, the last thought before meditation: last thoughts before death colour the whole of the consciousness. So if our last thought is God, Christ, the angels, we will raise our consciousness, but if it is our jewellery or a large plate of roast beef we will be pulled down into matter.

Life is but a continual process of change, a procession of births and deaths which are, like everything else, complementary opposites. Birth and death are bridges which are closely linked. If, for example, you have a difficult birth it will usually follow that you will be terrified of death. Ultimately, there should be no birth and no death, only continuity: an uninterrupted flow of being.

It takes many lives to work out our difficulties so that we can find this essential unity. Life after life we search for ourselves until finally we can see our whole journey from beginning to end. We realize the completeness of ourselves, the integration of the whole self, in every life and the wisdom beyond. Our mission on earth will have been accomplished.

As healers, then, we have to be able to transform people. We have to create in them the ability to reach out for their highest aspirations. We are not here merely to make organs function better. There are larger issues at stake. Healing is meant to change the patient and, if necessary, his way of life. We are here to allow the patient to raise his consciousness, to help him understand that earth is a school in which he is meant to learn his lessons and to work out his karma. He may have come for a special purpose and the healing is meant to help him realize his vocation.

Appendix I: Exercises and Meditations

Stretching Exercises for Releasing Tension from the Physical Body

Sit in a chair and make yourself comfortable. Relax your hands on the arms of the chair. If the chair is armless let them fall on either side or, if you prefer, you can put them in your lap. Now stretch your legs out directly in front of you and become aware of your feet. Start by moving the toes of both feet slowly backwards and forwards, allowing freedom of movement in that area. Notice if any of the toes do not move uniformly. Next, move both feet backwards and forwards as much as possible, bending them from the ankle joints. Repeat this from six to ten times, either separately or both together. Next point the feet, then raise the toes as strongly as you can. Bend the feet at the ankles bringing them up towards you as far as you can (which stretches the calves) and try to push the toes down away from you without moving the ankles. Repeat this from six to ten times. Next, do some ankle rotations. Keeping the rest of the body very relaxed rotate the right foot clockwise, then do the same thing anti-clockwise and repeat this with the left leg about six to ten times. Always rest a little after each series of exercises. Close your eyes for about half a minute and rest. Now rotate the knees, first to the right then to the left. Then put your foot back gently on the floor. Now, turn your attention to the hands. Hold the arms straight in front of your body so that they are on a horizontal plane from the shoulders. Stretch and tense the fingers of both hands, then close the fingers over the thumb and make a tight fist. Again stretch and open, tensing the fingers from six to ten times. Bend the hands at the wrist as if you are pressing the palms against the wall. Now bend the hands down from the wrist and point the fingers downwards, repeating from six to ten times. Clench the right fist and rotate it clockwise ten times, then anti-clockwise. Repeat the same treatment with the left hand. Extend both hands in front of the body with the fingers clenched and rotate the wrists together. Try to sense the tension in the hands, always relaxing well when you have finished the series of exercises. Stretch the hands forward then bend at the elbows and bring the hands back to the shoulders and do this several times, stretching and bending. Make a circular movement from the shoulder joints keeping the fingers in contact with the shoulders. Try to make the movement of each elbow as large as possible, bringing the elbows in contact with each other in front of the chest as you rotate. Now think about the neck. This is a place where tension accumulates very easily. Place the hands on the lap and gently allow the head to tilt to one side, then roll it towards the shoulder, turning it to the right first, moving it round and letting it drop at the back and then over to the opposite shoulder and forwards. Try to do this in a very relaxed way. There are different ways of breathing while you do this. You can take a breath as you move the head round, breathing out as your head comes down. It is always good to yawn as the head goes round. Some people like to breathe in halfway until the head drops to the back and breathe out as they bring it forward. When you have done this think of the eyes. Close them, facing towards the sun, rub the palms of the hands together and place them over your eyes. Repeat this often during the day, particularly if your eyes are troubling you.

The following stretching exercises are done lying on the ground, so find a comfortable place free from draughts. The aim, first of all, is to stretch and align the spine so that all parts will eventually touch the ground. It may be necessary for you to place a thin book under your neck to get the correct alignment. Gradually you will be able to do away with the book. For the second exercise place your legs about eighteen inches apart and raise your arms so that they rest flat on the floor above your head, making the grail shape. Notice how far your shoulders are from the ground and whether they are at different heights off the floor. For this it is helpful to have a friend to watch and inform you. As tension is released your shoulders will come closer to the floor, your back will lengthen and your chin will naturally re-align. For the third exercise lower your arms slightly so that they stretch out on a horizontal plane with the shoulders. Draw up your feet so that the soles are flat on the floor and gradually let your knees open outwards, responding to the natural pull of gravity. If you persist with this exercise they will gradually fall lower and lower. Fourth exercise: leaving your arms at shoulder level slowly roll your hips to the right side, letting your legs curl up like an embryo in the womb, simultaneously bringing your head to the left. Return to the centre keeping your lower spine in contact with the floor and repeat the movement on the other side. Gradually each knee should fit into the arch of the opposite leg. Do not be downhearted if at first this is not the case. As you persist you will become supple. Fifth exercise: roll on your left side and bring your right knee across, keeping it on the ground by holding it with your left hand. Starting at the knee gently try to sweep your right arm up, keeping it extended and trying to maintain contact with the floor. As you reach the top of your head roll over so that the shoulders are as flat as possible on the floor and your right arm is stretched above your head, then bring it down the right side, always keeping it fully extended, and back again round to the knee. Then do the same thing lying on your right side. If you find that your arm is considerably far from the floor it will take a little time to correct and for you to become supple, so do this exercise very gently. Sixth exercise: lie flat on your back relaxing as deeply as you can. Start to raise one leg slowly, as high as you can go. Now bend the knee and bring it down as far as possible towards the chest. Place your hands around it and see how far you can bring it towards your body. Raise your forehead and if possible bring it to the knee. Relax and lie back, then repeat with the other leg, going through the whole sequence for two or three minutes. If you are unable to bring your knee all the way down to the chest do persist with this exercise. It will protect you from lower back troubles later and you will get a splendid feeling of lengthening over the whole body.

For the final exercise kneel on the ground, sitting back on the heels in order to stretch the back. Now push your hands out in front of you and stretch forward like a cat, lower your buttocks and bring your hands to lie at the sides of your feet. Bring the top of your head down in front of your knees. Rest a moment then bring your hands forward and place them, one palm on top of the other. Rest your forehead on top. Close your eyes and relax. This is an excellent way to relieve stress at the end of the day. It is also good for alleviating lower back problems and encouraging energies to rise up the spine, flooding the mind and body with vitality.

Breathing Exercises

Breathing exercises are excellent for concentrating and balancing the mind. They can either relax the body or recharge it with energy depending on how the exercises are practised. Here is an example. Start with the mind in the middle of the forehead and breathe in, moving the attention round the head. Then breathe out and relax. Do this exercise three times to the right and three times to the left. Then take the mind over the forehead, down the back of the head, through the neck, under the chin, through the nostrils and back into the forehead, all on the in-breath. Do this three times going backwards, three times going forwards. For relaxation you concentrate on the out-breath: as your breathe out you imagine draining all the tension out of the brain. For recharging you concentrate on the in-breath: as you breathe in you concentrate on drawing clear fresh energies into the brain.

Another Recharging Exercise

Lie down with your head towards the north and breathe in gold through the top of the head all the way down to the feet. Then breathe out silver, starting with the feet and going up to the top of the head again. Repeat this seven times.

The following exercise will ensure that all parts of your body are linked up. First, you breathe in, taking your mind from the sole of the foot up into the knee, three times, relaxing on the out-breath; then three times from the knee to the hip and into the base chakra; three times from the base chakra to the abdomen, three times from abdomen to solar plexus, three times from solar plexus to heart. Now transfer your attention to your fingers and breathe from the fingers to the elbows three times, three times from the elbows to the shoulders, three times from throat to third eye.

The following is an opening and expanding exercise. Hold both hands over the base centre and breathe in. As you breathe out stretch your hands to the extremities of your auric space, keeping them at the level of the base centre. Repeat this three times. You do this with all the centres, breathing in and then, every time on the out-breath, stretching your arms out at the level of the chakra you are working with. When you get to the third eye just concentrate while breathing in, do not touch the forehead. Then, forming a chalice with your hands, concentrate on the top of the head. At the end of the exercise you can place your hands in the prayer position over the head, then draw them down over the forehead, over the lips and the heart and so on, closing up the energies in this way.

Counting the breath is a useful exercise for balancing and concentrating. When we breathe and count, it is like taking steps in our consciousness. It is possible to descend into the basement of our being by moving down in colour steps. As we breathe into the red centre, for example, we can use this as an exercise for exploring and releasing all the anger, desires and needs, letting go of any frustration to do with sexual relationships. We can step up to the orange, breathe in and try to let go of all the things we are too involved in. Perhaps we are inclined to eat too much and too often, perhaps we need to collect possessions and to hold on to physical things, rely on friends. We have to look at and try to let go of all the habits and needs we have of the tangible things in life. On the yellow ray there are all the mental

145

habits, the links with the mind, the need for the mind to possess ideas and concepts. On the heart ray we might look at our relationships, trying not to be involved just with one person, one animal, but endeavouring to embrace the Whole and link with the universal consciousness. On the blue we might try to get rid of saying things that are not necessary – all those things that link with the voice. Perhaps we praise someone because we want something out of them, or we bombard people with our miseries and problems which really we could resolve by ourselves. These are all vocal things which we sometimes have to work to get rid of. Eventually we must reach the stage where we do not hold on to anything. We have to release all things. Holding on at whatever level interferes with our flow of energy.

The Principles of Visualization and Guided Meditations

Any visualization, or guided meditation, should contain some essential ingredients. Here, as an example, is a simple meditation containing all the necessary archetypal patterns. You imagine a great golden sun above your head. A shaft of light descends in which you can see steps, a golden ladder is climbing up to the sun. Climb up this ladder of light, find the door, open it and go through. Now you are in a temple. In front of you see a large stone altar on which there is a crystal goblet, or cup, full of the sparkling, clear waters of life. You sit here quietly for a little while, then you pick up the cup and drink from the waters of life. So you should start with the idea of taking a journey, carrying only those things which are absolutely necessary. You can go through a field of corn, find yourself in a sunny meadow beside a stream. Here there is a tree which changes colours with the seasons. You can notice mountains in the distance. Your surroundings should always be warm, safe and beautiful and it is important that there is the idea of rising up. You might see a beautiful white building with steps leading up to the door. You climb up the steps and go in and find yourself in a magnificent library lined with golden books, thus creating a link between beauty, wisdom and gold. You can create a little desk perhaps and sit down and review your life or your day. Another way is to go into a room and there is a little easel and you imagine painting yourself, feeling the colours, the clothes you would like to wear, the setting in which you would like to be. If it's a garden or a room you can explore it, you can explore the consciousness of that particular place. Remember, though, that in certain kinds of meditation people can get very uncomfortable exploring this kind of consciousness because what they are doing is exploring themselves. Sometimes it's better that they should do this in a group or under the supervision of someone who is experienced. If we approach the attic we are approaching a consciousness that is going up and if we go into a cellar we can bring up to the light all kinds of old things. Remember too that when we go into rooms or houses we must always close doors behind us. We always need to know what we are doing. To end the meditation it is good to guide people into a garden where they see flowers of various shades: red flowers, orange flowers, yellow flowers and so on, and in the middle there might be a cleansing fountain. Always bring yourself, your patient or your group back through the body, earthing yourselves, being aware of the limbs and especially the feet. It is a good idea to have a cup of tea and really come down to earth before going home.

The following are suggestions: guidelines for relaxation and visualization exercises. You can put them on tape or, keeping to the principles, you can adapt them and compose your own.

Relaxation Exercise

It is a good idea to start any relaxation exercise with the cleansing breath (p. 157). Imagine that the space around you has various levels of awareness and that if you breathe up the back of the body from the heels to the top of the head and breathe out down the front of the body this awareness will grow and you will sense the space around you. Feel the differences and make sure that the left and the right side, the back and the front of the body are uniform as far as the aura is concerned. So once you have breathed up the back and down the front seven times, moving with each breath away from the body, do the same thing seven times up the right side and down the left.

Now place your mind on the forehead and try to feel that the energies which are going to relax the base of the body are gathering there. Imagine that this area feels much stronger now, that you are confident that whatever comes through you will take away any restrictions you may feel at the base of the body. So begin with the toes. Take your mind and place it in your toes. Imagine that this area is very slowly being taken over. Very deeply plunge your thoughts into your toes so that a great sense of well-being goes into the feet. Try to feel that the feet are beginning to melt a little and that you can feel yourself massage them, very gently moving your mind between the toes. Impregnate the feet, deeply submerge yourself into them. The feet become bigger, maybe a little heavier and then gradually try to see whether you can make them feel transparent. Imagine the contours of the feet disappearing and there is just an empty space. It is all very quiet, all very still. Your feet are going to be more relaxed than they have ever been before. Then slowly allow your mind to wander higher, feel yourself moving gently into the bone structure and like a soft wave move upwards until you reach your knees. Submerge yourself into your knees. Try to think of your knees like two deep pools. Place your thoughts into these pools and try to feel a deep sense of well-being and relaxation moving within the knees themselves. They feel warm. The legs feel longer. Very slowly and gently they start to become transparent all the way up to the knees. Then the knees start to disappear and your legs are no longer a part of you. Somewhere within the structure you let go. There is no more holding on. There is an enormous sense of well-being and freedom as you encompass the thighs. There, within the deep structure of the thighs you stretch. Try to feel your mind stretching inside your thighs. Try to feel that they are transparent, translucent, so that you can see inside, you can see all the nerves, all the vessels. You can feel the blood moving. You can sense your bones and within the thighs a lovely sense of well-being. No matter what memories

148

there are here, the way you feel now, the way your legs feel is going to be the only thing that will count. The energy purifies and clears the old memory patterns. This flowing red energy is like a warm blanket around you. If there are parts of you that are always cold, parts that never seem right and need the warmth of this red energy let it flow into those parts now. Produce some of your own warmth and try to feel it. Try to feel it even in your toes so that you can sense the energy restoring whatever is lacking in your body.

Now go into your abdomen. The more you relax this area, the easier it will absorb the goodness from your food. Think of your organs, of the different sounds they make, how they all compensate for each other. Try to feel that the organs are going to have a wonderful peaceful feeling. Make the abdomen transparent. Pour yourself inside, try to feel the richness and depth of your giving. Do not have any boundaries. Think of that energy and how you need it, think that this energy provides so much for the activity of the body and mind. So if you need any orange anywhere just let it travel and move wherever necessary. This may make you feel a little more active. Activity in a relaxed body is quite healthy. So try to feel this energy and try to sense it. It is very warm and rather sunny and when this energy moves around you feel a kind of glow. It is not as warm as the red energy but there is a nice friendly glow about it. Imagine that you are looking into a fire and seeing the reds and oranges flickering there and try to think of the warmth, the feeling of pleasure in your organs as they relax and that energy allows itself to be free of any thought patterns. As we move higher we come to the solar plexus – the area that gathers energy for the left side of the brain. It is a very special area, holding something sunny and bright. If you relax you can remember all the golden days in your life, the golden sunny days, lying perhaps on a beach, walking in a garden, kissing somebody you love. Perhaps your body lacks the sun, perhaps you do not have a sunny disposition, perhaps you need this golden yellow in your life. Try to relax to this golden feeling so deeply you can get immersed in it and the gold is set free right through the body. You can feel streams of sunshine in every pore so that the sunny aspect becomes alive in the body. As this area relaxes more and more you find that you are naturally gathering energy so that, even though you may have relaxed, these warm bright energies have penetrated your being and you feel very content. You have a lovely sense of well-being in these centres. So now, having relaxed the bottom three centres try to move all the way back down to the feet again and have the feeling that this area is well stretched, that the circulation has improved, that the well-being in this area has gone higher and the base of the body is now relaxing quite deeply.

So now you can pay attention to the most vulnerable part of all, which is the heart. Begin with your hands. Once you have let go completely everything you touch, everything that you feel with your hands will help you to release the heart centre. Place the mind on the fingertips and feel that there is a natural flow of energies here. Try to see what you are doing with your hands. Try to feel that you are putting a great depth of relaxation into the palms of your hands and imagine yourself going into the fingers and travelling deep into the palms. Sometimes life is difficult and we hold on to people, things and ideas, things that we should let go. So try to let go, not just on the surface level but on a really deep level. Allow the strength of your mind to prevail until your hands feel almost translucent and invisible. Try to feel that there are no contours to your fingers so that your hands feel totally rested and at peace. Then allow the consciousness to travel upwards to penetrate through the bone structure deeply into the nervous system and imagine your hands getting longer. Bathe your elbows, massage them with your mind, saturate them with your thoughts. Try to make sure the flow goes through them. Go a little higher and move right through the shoulders and measure from the tip of the fingers all the way to the shoulders and feel there is a flow. Try to sense if there are any blockages. Then with your imagination try to feel that your energy flow is so deep, so penetrating, so real, that nothing stands in its way. Try to visualize that the energy flow seems to be getting easier, that you are stronger and better. Imagine that your spine is going to allow all the nerves to rest and that somewhere within your nervous system there is going to be a strange peace, a nice, restful dreamy peace. The muscles of the spine begin to let go. Submerge yourself at the base of the spine, almost like a diver diving into a tunnel and feel yourself moving gently, a sense of well-being flowing through your spine. Try to feel your consciousness moving slowly up the spine. As it flows you can feel the spine getting longer, that you are stretched and a sense of depth and penetration seems to be here.

Imagine now that your consciousness is a little boat, with white sails, sailing slowly up the spine. Imagine that you are sitting in the boat, looking at the shore with its green trees and soft grasses. Take the boat close to the shore, look at the green and feel all those lovely green colours that are part of your heart. Your heart feels nice and warm now. Lovely warm energies are here, the rose of spiritual love is glowing and you feel very comfortable. You are relaxing the heart muscles deeply and you feel your circulation flowing inside your body. All the things that have troubled your heart have melted away, there is an enormous sense of freedom and the sense of well-being moves up the body. The back of the neck loosens and any constrictions you have felt here gradually melt away. Now you can relax your chin. Sense that you are going deeper into its structure, that the tongue is relaxing very deeply and that you can go inside the throat and relax that. Relax the roof of the palate. Try to feel the breath going into the nostrils. Imagine the breath as nectar and, as you drink, strength and peace flows into your body. Relax around the ears and then go into your eyes. Try to imagine that you can still see although your eyes are closed. You can see the room, you can see yourself lying down, you can see your face and your eyes. Go deep inside the eyes and allow them to relax very deeply. Try to feel that you are relaxing the forehead. Imagine you are standing by a window, that the curtains are closed. Imagine that you are very relaxed and dreamy, you have just woken up and are very sleepy still. Gradually the curtains become more and more invisible and you are looking into the windows of your mind. Imagine that you are looking inside, the mind becomes very peaceful and is completely relaxed. Here in the peacefulness of your mind you see a little chapel on the hill, or perhaps a pagoda in the garden. You find somewhere you can form and visualize a place of rest and refuge, a place where no thoughts can penetrate.

You have taken a journey right through the body and you have reached this point at which you can allow yourself to sit quietly. You feel cleaner, more relaxed, more contented than ever before. Try to feel you are translucent now and that the body does not have any hard contours at all. Just sit there and relax.

When you are ready gradually move various parts of yourself. Move your face and your shoulders, your torso, your legs and hands. Through gentle movements come back to reality.

Exercise for Making a Healing Fountain

Let us begin by making ourselves very comfortable and through our feet earthing ourselves well. So relax the feet and the toes and let us try to have no memories here. The aspect of walking does not exist in the consciousness. We are not holding on to paths or roads, we have only our inner path, our inner road. Release and allow the arms to rest and try to see that our hands have no memories of holding. No longer do we need our physical hands. So rest the hands, rest the shoulders. Rest every part of the body, releasing the tension so that our organs inside us are bathed in a warm gold light. Go into the lungs and try to feel the breath of all things so that the lungs feel part of the harmony of the universe. Let us imagine that, although we are still sitting here, we can go from level to level of awareness. Imagine that we are standing in a corridor. At the end of this corridor there is a light and as we go towards the light we feel a beautiful feeling of opening out. The air vibrates as we touch it so that our own vibrations feel heightened. We are standing on a mosaic floor, a floor that is different from any other floor. The colours vibrate and there is a lovely feeling as the colours penetrate through our feet. As we walk we feel that we can see everything and that we are everywhere, we are not limited to the space we are in. Our eyes seem to penetrate

152

and see enormous distances and our whole body seems to feel that the space around it is much fresher. As we walk forward we become aware that this beautiful mosaic pathway is leading towards a great domed building. It is so pure and white that it is dazzling and as we approach we know we are welcome. Someone in a white robe is waiting to meet us. We feel his presence before we reach the spot where he stands. Imagine that he guides us into a hall so large and spacious we seem to float rather than walk. Everywhere there is light. We sense that we are approaching a place of miracles, a place of healing fountains. We walk through a magnificent room in which there is a fountain. The force of this fountain cascading in a rainbow fills the whole room. Millions of vibratory rays pour down like coloured drops of water. Imagine our energies, our auras, flowing like this fountain. Sense the movements round us, round our faces, in front and behind us. All thoughts dissolve and a kind of strange freshness fills the space. Let us walk towards the fountain and hold out our hands and try to gather a little of this energy and see how it feels, try to see that there are pools of it around. It is floating and flowing everywhere. Now feel that beside us are all the people who are on our list and we draw them into the fountain so that they become part of it. We are giving all these people strength and healing from the fountain. (At this point you can read the list of names, but do not mention the illness as this would create a negative thoughtform.) Now let us imagine that all round this building there are corridors of colour, beautiful corridors each one vibrating to a different colour shade. Let us see which colour draws us, whether we are drawn to the warm colours, whether we need to go to the greens, the blues, the violets, the purples, or just towards white light. Let us move down the corridor, the one we have chosen, and try to feel the space around us pouring that colour into our being. The corridor may be long and as we continue down the tunnel of our own consciousness we find lights appear in the distance as though a new dawn is breaking. Through the soft mists, through the gentle light, we feel ourselves going deeper and deeper and we enter into bright light. As we walk out everything is shimmering. We are seeing life as it really is. Flowers are radiating strongly, they look almost as if they are made of crystals. They shimmer and they glow. The ground is radiating. Everything seems to have a beautiful radiance. Stay still for a moment and feel this lovely radiance. But every journey has to have a homecoming and now, having released all the tiredness, all the illness, all the unhappiness that we have collected through our lives, we feel that we are stronger and richer and we can come back. Let us return again down the colour tunnel and go back to the fountain. Move away and go out of the building, returning once more down the mosaic path, gradually sensing the feet, the hands, the limbs. Now let us relax and rest and enjoy the peace and when we are ready we can open our eyes.

All these exercises are suggestions for you to expand and develop, to use in the way that is best for you. You may feel that it would be appropriate for you to make tapes of your visualisation exercises so that you can follow them in meditation.

Appendix II: Guidance Notes

The following is the suggested procedure for meetings, reproduced with permission from the guidance notes of the National Federation of Spiritual Healers.

The meeting room should be arranged with a small table in the middle, on which a candle or flowers or a plant has been placed, and chairs placed around it in a circle.

Opening
The Great Invocation or other prayer of protection and invocation is read by the group leader or a selected member; alternatively, all may join in The Great Invocation while a member lights a candle. (The Great Invocation is given at the end of this section.)

Members are advised to prepare themselves for the relaxation and attunement that follows by stretching the body, raising the arms upwards, sideways and forward and to use the cleansing breath (p. 157) to clear away negativity and help create spiritual protection and an atmosphere of stillness and peace within the group. Members link hands for about a minute, giving love with the right hand and receiving peace with the left. This act serves to bring the group together so that they can receive and radiate the maximum amount of healing energy.

Grounding or earthing
It is necessary to ensure that everyone is safely grounded and relaxed before attempting to raise the consciousness. Members should turn their attention to their bodies – legs uncrossed, back as straight as possible and supported if

necessary, hands resting comfortably in the lap, focusing first on the feet and feeling them rooted in the ground.

Relaxing
The group leader guides the others by helping them to be conscious of their breathing, helping them to breathe in and out gently without forcing the breath in any way, releasing (on the out-breath) tension and stress from feet, ankles, calves, thighs, buttocks, front and back of body, hands and arms, head, face, neck and shoulders. The physical relaxation completed, attention is again focused on the breath, breathing in peace and breathing out love. These thoughts help to still and raise the mind. Members can then visualize themselves as being centred within a circle of golden light in preparation for a guided visualization.

Visualization
It is helpful for a visualization to be developed by the group leader with the aim of bringing light into the body and converting it to a stream of pure energy radiating light from the heart into the centre of the group. The intention is to focus the energy into the centre of the group to build up a point of light, a centre of energy which is characteristically loving and healing.

Distant healing
A member first reads aloud a distant healing prayer and then the names on the healing list. Names have vibrations and each person is thus linked to the healing energies emanating from the centre of the group. Illnesses are not mentioned as these create negative thoughtforms. The group should operate to release a loving healing energy from the heart and through the mind, seeing it as a beam of light reaching out to each person who has asked for help.

The understanding behind this action is that the energy will be absorbed by the patient without interfering in any way with his free will. He can either receive it or reject it. It makes no difference whether the patient has asked for distant healing or whether the request has been made by a friend or relative without the patient's knowledge. It is recommended that the names remain on the list no longer than one month unless a further request is received.

The group leader must close the proceedings by bringing the group back to the level of physical consciousness. Members are asked first to focus their attention on their feet, feeling them firmly rooted on the ground, then to become aware of their bodies seated in the chairs. Everyone should feel centred and secure before opening their eyes, rubbing their hands together and stretching.

The Great Invocation
From the point of Light within the Mind of God
Let light stream forth into the minds of men.
Let Light descend on Earth.

From the point of Love within the Heart of God
Let Love stream forth into the hearts of men.
May Love return to Earth.

From the centre where the Will of God is known
Let purpose guide the little wills of men –
The purpose which the Masters know and serve.

From the centre which we call the race of men
Let the Plan of Love and Light work out
And may it seal the door where evil dwells.

Let Light and Love and Power restore the Plan on Earth.

The cleansing breath
This is an excellent breathing exercise which helps to strengthen and purify the energy-field around the body. It may be practised daily, preferably early in the morning and late in the evening and before meditation. It may also be used after healing treatment and should be taught to patients so that they may contribute to their own recovery.

Imagine you are like the yolk inside an egg and that between you and the shell are seven other layers. In other words, around the physical body you have seven invisible layers. On the *in-breath* imagine the breath moving up the back of the body from the feet to the top of the head. On the *out-breath* picture the breath moving down the front of the body and sweeping underneath the feet. Repeat seven times each time on the *in-breath* imagining the movement of the breath being a little further away from the body. On reaching the seventh in-breath you will be sweeping a wide circle in front and behind the body. You decide how far from the body each circle moves. There is no standard distance. Next repeat the process by imagining the breath moving up the right-hand side of the body from the feet to the top of the head on the in-breath and down the left-hand side of the body on the out-breath, again in the same way sweeping under the feet and moving away from the body in an ever-widening circle. Let go on the out-breath, releasing all the tension, stress and poisons from the body. Do not force the breath but aim to get the time taken for the in-breath and the out-breath to be the same, in other words, so that both breaths are more or less of the same length.

Index